SMART FOOD
FOR SMART KIDS

WITHDRAWN

Family Place Collection
Funded by the Carpenter Grant

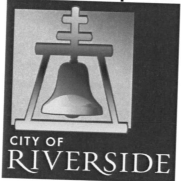

CITY OF
RIVERSIDE

Riverside Public Library

Other books by Patrick Holford from Piatkus:

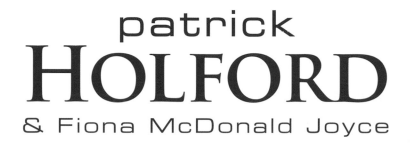

patrick
HOLFORD
& Fiona McDonald Joyce

SMART FOOD FOR SMART KIDS

Easy recipes to boost your child's health and IQ

piatkus

PIATKUS

First published in Great Britain in 2007 by Piatkus Books
Reprinted 2010

A CIP catalogue record for this book
is available from the British Library.

ISBN 978-0-7499-5345-4

Photograph credits
Chineham Park Primary School photos by Catherine Morgan: pp. 9, 37, 85;
photos by Nick Morris: pp. 45, 74, 129, 146; photos by Robin Matthews: pp. 41, 43,
56, 138, 144; p. 11 photo courtesy of Patrick Holford; p. 48 Getty Images/White
Rock; p. 78 Getty Images/Siri Stafford; p. 93 Getty Images/Greg Elms; p. 119 Getty
Images/Pat LaCroix; p. 132 Getty Images/George Doyle.

Text design by Nicky Barneby @ Barneby Ltd
Data manipulation by 4word Ltd, Bristol
Printed and bound in Italy by LEGO SpA

Piatkus
An imprint of
Little, Brown Book Group
100 Victoria Embankment
London EC4Y 0DY

An Hachette UK Company
www.hachette.co.uk

www.piatkus.co.uk

Contents

To Annabel Ray, Fiona's beautiful new niece.
May you be happy and healthy.

Acknowledgements

A huge thank you to all of the children and parents who tested recipes for this book, including Cricket Green school in Mitcham, Chineham Park Primary School in Basingstoke, the Alpert family (especially Erin and Joe), Manoj and Mukund Pujari, Hope Putt and Fiona's 'nearly nephews' Carl and Tom. Particular thanks must go to Marion and John Burgess in Caundle Marsh, and their children Lewis, Shelley and Paige, who not only tested lots of recipes but also gave very helpful and honest feedback and who have since converted to eating 'smart food' all the time! Thank you also to Catherine Morgan and Nick Morris, for taking such lovely photos of our children, to Deborah Colson, Sarah Hanson, and Jo Brooks, our brilliant and punctilious editor, who has worked tirelessly to produce another beautiful book.

Conversions used in the book

Dry measurements

Metric (g/kg)	Imperial (oz/lb)
25g	1oz
50g	2oz
75g	3oz
115g	4oz
125g	$4\frac{1}{2}$oz
140g	5oz
175g	6oz
200g	7oz
225g	8oz/$\frac{1}{2}$lb
250g	9oz
275g	$9\frac{3}{4}$oz
280 g	10 oz
300g	$10\frac{1}{2}$oz
325g	$11\frac{1}{2}$oz
350g	12oz
375g	13oz
400g	14oz
425g	15oz
450g	16oz/1lb

Liquid measurements

Metric (ml/litres)	Imperial (fl oz/pints)
30ml	1fl oz
60ml	2fl oz
90ml	3fl oz
120ml	4fl oz
150ml	5fl oz/$\frac{1}{4}$ pint
180ml	6fl oz
210ml	7fl oz
240ml	8fl oz
270ml	9fl oz
300ml	10fl oz/$\frac{1}{2}$ pint
330ml	11fl oz
360ml	12fl oz
390ml	13fl oz
420ml	14fl oz
450ml	15fl oz/$\frac{3}{4}$ pint
480ml	16fl oz
600ml	20fl oz/1 pint

Part 1
by Patrick Holford

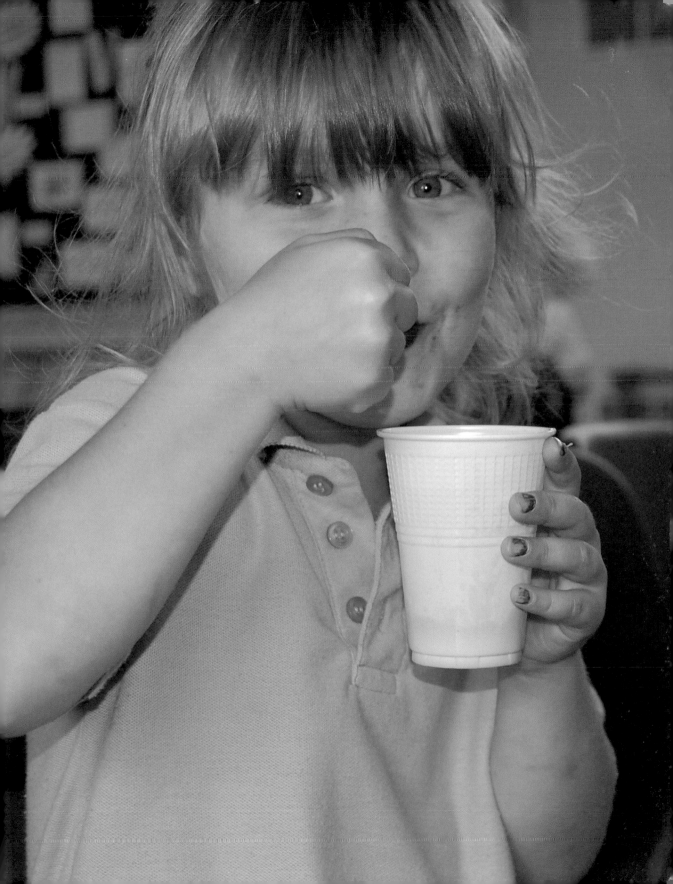

Introduction

You are probably already aware of the effect that certain foods (sugary snacks, for example) have on your child's behaviour, intelligence, happiness and health. Healthy eating is the single most important gift that you can give your child – and yourself. I guarantee that as you work through our recommendations in this book you will discover the benefits of feeding your child 'smart food'. The book has been developed for children over five years, but is also suitable for teenagers and you the parents, as well as younger toddlers (see the Start Early note on page 48).

When we met George he was often extremely defiant and had frequent stand-up rows with his mother. But since changing his diet and taking supplements he is a very different George, according to his mum. 'We no longer argue and it's a joy to take him out because his temper doesn't flare. The entire household is calmer. His sleep is much better too. It used to be difficult to get him to bed. Now he's going to bed much earlier (he often takes himself off to bed at 8pm) and going to sleep and sleeping right through.'

Leanne, who suffers from autism and used to be very shy and withdrawn, with daily tantrums, has changed dramatically. 'Her mood is so much better. She's much more communicative and even got up and sang Karaoke in the hotel when we were on holiday. I couldn't believe it,' says her mum, Margaret.

'He used to be aggressive. Now he's much calmer and even says sorry when he loses his temper. This never happened before,' said Sharon P., mother of Reece with quite profound ADHD (attention deficit and hyperactivity disorder).

Shaun's father Matt says, 'His schoolwork has improved dramatically in just a few weeks since we changed his diet and got him on the supplements. In fact, all four of our children are much calmer and more co-operative these days. It's great for them and also for my wife and me.'

These are the comments of some of the parents who took part in our Food for the Brain school projects in which we worked with parents, teachers and school caterers to improve children's nutrition, and then had the results measured independently. We've seen obvious improvements in the children's ability to maximise their potential, whether they were top or bottom of the class, or coping with disabilities such as autism.

We've written this book because we want to share the recipes and healthy-eating guidelines that produced such dramatic improvements. We want parents everywhere – whether your children have educational difficulties or not – to benefit from our experience. All children have a right to be nourished so that they can achieve to the best of their ability. Providing smart food for your kids needn't be complicated, and in this book we show you how to do it.

Because your child's brain and nutritional

needs are similar to an adult's, everything we recommend for your child is ideal for you, too. Countless sceptical mums and resistant dads have changed their diets to support their child through our Food for the Brain projects. As reported on *GMTV* and *Tonight with Trevor Macdonald* they have found their energy, mood and concentration soar as their unwanted weight falls away.

Make the smart choice – do it for yourself, and do it for your child. Transform the way your family eats, experience the benefits for yourself and see them in your children. Break free from the cultural conditioning and clever marketing that has created a disastrous diet we've been brought up to know and love, but which is, quite frankly, unfit for human consumption.

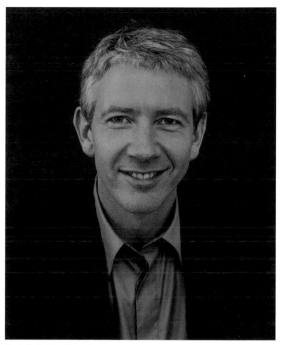

Patrick Holford

The future for an unhealthy society

* More than one-third of girls and one-fifth of boys will be obese by 2020.[1]
* There has been a 500 per cent increase in the number of prescriptions written for ADHD since 1991, and prescriptions keep rising.[2]
* ADHD affects 1 in 20 children in the UK (that's half a million children) and the incidence is rising.[3]
* A survey of children in London published in the *Lancet* finds that the incidence of autistic spectrum disorders has more than doubled in the last 20 years and now affects 1 in 86 children and, at least 1 in 50 boys.[4]

We may be criticised by some experts and scientists who say that we don't yet have all the proof of the power of 'optimum nutrition' – and to an extent this is true. There's been a desperate shortage of funds to carry out proper research into the effects of poor nutrition, largely because it's not in the interests of the food industry, who make billions from selling junk food. Nor is it in the interests of the pharmaceutical industry, which funds most medical research and makes huge profits from prescribing stimulant drugs such as Ritalin to the ever-increasing number of 'ADHD' children, currently one quarter of a million of whom are on a prescription. The government is only now starting to fund research after pressure from people such as chef and TV personality Jamie Oliver, organisations such as Food for the Brain Foundation and the tireless scientists who've been banging the drum for over a decade.

However, existing research certainly supports our recommendations. None of the healthy-eating suggestions and supplements we recommend is in any way dangerous. If you had seen the transformations in children that we've seen, you'd understand why we want to shout about it from the rooftops and help parents put these simple food principles into practice.

If you want a healthy future for your children, now is the time to act. Eating smart food is not difficult or boring, it doesn't take more time or cost more money – it's simply what human beings are designed to eat. One mother, Nicola, said, 'This is now my way of life. I cannot think of a single reason to go back to what I used to eat'.

Parents would tell us: 'My child just won't eat vegetables'. But by the time Fiona had finished cooking with them and giving them new things to taste, the children were asking for these new foods.

This book is designed not only as a cookbook but also as a way to get your child involved in cooking and learning about food, and we have highlighted the recipes that are easy for children to help with. This is smart food for smart kids and parents.

Wishing you the best of health,

Patrick Holford

Tried-and-tested recipes

I want to introduce you to Fiona McDonald Joyce, our 'kitchen wizard'. Fiona trained with me as a nutritional therapist and, through her love of food, learned how to make optimum nutrition simple to prepare and delicious to eat. She's worked with hundreds of children and parents in our Food for the Brain Schools Campaign.

SMART FOOD AT SCHOOL

If you want to transform your child's diet, in addition to feeding your child the best quality food at home, you need to think about their food at school. For this reason we worked with the educational charity, Food for the Brain Foundation (see page 151), to start a schools campaign.

Our aim is to help parents and teachers to understand the power of nutritious food and to use food and supplements to:

* Improve children's attention, language and learning
* Improve children's emotional stability (fewer outbursts, and less compulsive behaviour and aggression)
* Improve children's physical co-ordination
* Improve children's health and happiness.

We want to create a sustainable 'smart food' culture at school that can be shared with other schools and families. We want to empower children to make the right choices.

We set out to achieve this by: providing healthy breakfasts, fruit, healthy snacks and water; improving school lunches and home meals; giving all children a multivitamin/mineral called Dinochews made by Higher Nature and an EyeQ essential fat supplement made by Equazen (see Product and Supplement Directory) and including structured exercise most days using a system called Speed Agility Quickness (SAQ). We helped transform the breakfast clubs and lunch menus, and ran workshops with the children and parents.

We've worked with two schools: Cricket Green in Merton, Surrey – a special educational needs school for children with difficulties such as autism and ADHD – and Chineham Park Primary School in Basingstoke, Hampshire, a school that was struggling to achieve acceptable SAT scores (the national measure of how kids at school are doing).

Each child was assessed by an educational psychologist before the nutritional programme began, and after three and seven months.

At the time of writing we can't give you final results of the Chineham Park kids as we're just a few months in. They'll be revealed on the television programme *Tonight with Trevor Macdonald*. However, already, some parents are noticing big improvements in their children's willingness to eat a wider variety of foods, their concentration and their behaviour.

Tommy's mother Katy has found that her six-year-old son is 'finding reading a lot easier these days'. She adds: 'It's not the struggle that it used to be and he's even wanting to read now which he never did before. He seems happier, with fewer tantrums, fighting less with his brother and more likely to do as he's told without argument.' Harry's mum Joan says, 'He's calmer, his writing is coming on well and his maths is much better.'

Other parents and teachers, and the children themselves, have also reported improvements. At the start of the Chineham School project we ran a Conners test on the children. This measures various aspects of behaviour and performance. We gave the children supplements and started to improve their diets, and then retested after seven months (the time we think it takes to really benefit from a smart food diet). The graphs below show improvement in every measure we made in those children who were having problems, rated by their teachers and their parents. Scores above 60 indicate problem behaviour.

The results at Cricket Green were even more spectacular. School meals have been transformed, thanks to Eden, the school caterers who installed a kitchen in the school and prepare healthy wholefoods on the premises. At snack time children can be seen nibbling on fruits and seeds. Gone are all sweets and sweetened drinks.

The parent ratings showed highly significant improvements as visible on the graph below. These include:

* A 15% reduction in defiant and oppositional behaviour
* An 18% reduction in anxiety and shyness
* A 25% reduction in psychosomatic symptoms such as headaches, tummy aches etc.

TEACHER RATINGS

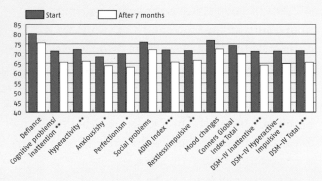

PARENT RATINGS

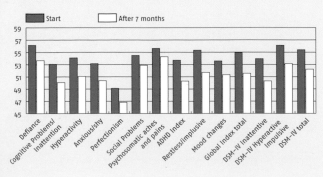

PARENT RATINGS

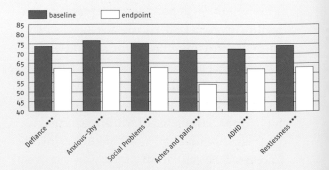

The factors with an asterisk (*) are those that had a significant improvement. The greater the number of asterisks, the more significant the improvement in that particular area. DSM is an abbreviation for Diagnostic and Statistical Manual – these ratings are used by doctors to diagnose mental health conditions.

Bear in mind that these are the 'average' improvement, so some children were doing much better than this. Scores above 60 indicate problem behaviour.

The teacher ratings showed significant improvements in restlessness and impulsiveness (5.6% reduction), inattention (9.3% reduction), hyperactivity and impulsivity (9.2% reduction), social problems (9% reduction) and anxiety and shyness (10% reduction).

Celia Dawson, Headteacher of Cricket Green school comments: 'The quality of school meals, packed lunches and snacks has improved. The most significant changes have been noticed in the younger pupils, probably because we are in a better position to influence their diet and eating habits. The changes we have seen fall into three main areas: improvements in the quality of communication and use of language, greater attention to tasks and therefore improved quality in work such as handwriting, and parents reporting changes in mood swings with pupils being calmer.'

Teacher Jenny Lloyd states: 'The children are more aware of healthy and unhealthy foods and the benefits of healthy eating now and they enjoy school dinners a lot more due to better quality of food.'

Celia Dawson adds: 'Having reached the end of the Food for the Brain Project I would say that its impact has been significant in a variety of ways and we have noticed changes in a number of our pupils, and parents have also noticed these. Some children are calmer and less active, therefore they are accessing the learning opportunities provided by our excellent staff. The consequence of this has been improvements in writing, communication, together with improved mood and social behaviour.'

Learning from the schools

We found that a number of parents and pupils were sceptical at first, but in time, they came to believe in the power of nutrition. The results aren't always immediate, so it's something you need to commit to for at least three months. When you begin eating smart food you'll be introduced to new foods and new ways to prepare them. It takes a bit of getting used to, but we can assure you that the results are worth it. The families we have introduced you to didn't do everything we recommended, they just did the best they could. That's all you need to do.

You too can take part in this project by following the advice in this book and by testing your child's diet and performance with a FREE on-line profile that gives personalised advice on simple changes to make to maximise your child's potential at www.foodforthebrain.org.

CHAPTER 1
How Food Builds the Brain

You can already see that we believe passionately in the important role that food plays in enabling children to fulfil their potential, both academically and socially. I'd like to give you the background information on how good nutrition can make such a difference to children.

Scientists studying behavioural problems and development in children today look at the mind and body as two separate parts. Few psychologists know much about brain chemistry and the importance of nutrition, and few doctors know enough about the psychological or nutritional factors that affect a child's development.

But it's not just the scientists who live by this misconception that mind and body are separate. It's all of us. It's undoubtedly second nature to you to help your child grow physically strong and healthy. But when they're having difficulty concentrating, behaving badly or struggling to read, does the thought that they might be poorly nourished cross your mind? If it doesn't, it's vital to know that all these attributes and behaviours depend on the food your child puts into his or her mouth.

Brain fats

Your brain is made from fat – in fact a whopping 60 per cent. Eating the right kinds of fats, called omega-3 and omega-6 fats, found in fish and seeds, makes you smarter. Eating the wrong kinds of fats, found in fried and processed foods, as well as too much poor-quality meat, literally makes the brain thicker, and they make you thicker too! So vital are these fats to the growing baby in the womb that it will literally rob its mother's brain to make its own – if a pregnant woman's diet is deficient in the essential fats, her brain will actually get smaller!

Brain energy

Your brain runs on glucose, the simple form of sugar. Too much makes you hyper and causes all kinds of problems, so balancing your child's blood sugar level, which is how glucose gets delivered to the brain, is vital for attention and focus. This means eating what are called low Glycemic Load, or low-GL foods. (See page 24 for more about this.)

Joined-up thinking

In the womb, a baby builds thousands of brain cells, called neurons, every minute. By the age of two, a child's brain has approximately 100 billion of them. That's about the same number of neurons as there are trees in the Amazon! And just like the interlocking branches of those rainforest trees, the neurons are connected up. So the brain is essentially a network of specialised nerve cells, all linked up to other neurons.

Protein – the messengers

The brain cells talk to each other by sending messages, delivered by messenger chemicals called neurotransmitters. These neuro-transmitters are made from protein. So this is an essential brain food. The message is sent from a sending station and received in a receiving station, called a receptor. These sending and receiving stations are built out of phospholipids (present in eggs and organ meats) and amino acids (the raw material of protein). Turning an amino acid into a neurotransmitter is no simple job. Enzymes in the brain that depend on vitamins, minerals and special amino acids accomplish this task.

Good nutrition starts from birth

At each stage of brain development, achieving optimum nutrition is essential to guarantee that your child achieves his or her full potential. At birth, the level of essential fats in the umbilical cord will give an indication of the child's speed of thinking at the age of eight. In eight-year-olds, the blood level of homocysteine (an amino acid that can indicate whether a child has high or low levels of B vitamins) will be linked to their school grades.[5] If a teenager's daily intake of zinc is just twice the level of the recommended daily allowance (RDA), this can improve attention and concentration to an astonishing degree.[6] And at any age, eating too much sugar and damaged fats has proved to have harmful effects on learning and behaviour.

From all this, you can see how the food your child eats builds the very structure of his or her brain, from the neurons themselves to the messages that shoot from one to another. So food governs how your child thinks and feels to a massive degree.

Essential brain foods

Optimum nutrition means achieving the right intake of all these essential brain foods:

* **Essential fats** Smart fats build smart brains.
* **A low-sugar and low-GL diet** To balance your child's blood sugar, the brain's superfuel.
* **Vitamins and minerals** The intelligent nutrients that keep the brain in tune.
* **Protein and amino acids** The brain's messengers.
* **Phospholipids** Memory molecules that give 'oomph' to the brain.

But this isn't the whole story. You will also need to avoid substances that damage the brain.

Foods to avoid

* **Damaged fats** From deep-fried food to hydrogenated fats found in most margarines as well as commercial cakes, biscuits and pastries.
* **Refined sugar** Carbohydrates, from white bread to sugar, robbed of essential nutrients.
* **Chemical food additives** Colourings, flavourings and preservatives.
* **Food allergens** Common foods your child might be allergic to.

The recipes in this book deliver all the key nutrients your child's brain (and our own) needs, and removes the bad guys. The next four chapters explain the four golden rules, which are:

 THE GOLDEN RULES

1 Ensure essential fats.
2 Eat a low-sugar and low-GL diet.
3 Increase vitamins and minerals.
4 Consider food allergies and chemical sensitivities.

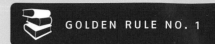

CHAPTER 2

Ensure Essential Fats

There are two kinds of essential fats, called omega-3 and omega-6 fats. Of these, the omega-3s that occur in fish oils are the more important for brain function. Plenty of studies have shown a clear benefit in children who take these as supplements on a daily basis. Although there is not the same level of scientific evidence to show that equivalent results can be achieved by eating oily fish, it stands to reason that including it in your child's diet is good news for his or her brain development.

We recommend eating oily fish two to three times a week, as well as eating seeds, which are another source of these essential fats, so Fiona has come up with plenty of child-friendly recipes to help you get these vital nutrients into your child. We also recommend taking supplements for these essential fats (see page 23 for recommended amounts).

Other sources of omega-3

One specific kind of omega-3 fat, called DHA, is vital for the developing brain, so it is especially important in pregnancy and infancy. Another kind, called EPA, has proven effective for improving poor attention, hyperactivity, depression and anxiety. Both EPA and DHA are found in fish oils. There is another type of omega-3 fat, called alpha-linolenic acid (ALA), which is found in foods of vegetable origin, such as flaxseeds (linseeds) and pumpkin seeds. Although beneficial, only a very small amount gets converted into the more powerful EPA and DHA, so it is best to obtain a direct source of EPA and DHA, either from eating fish or taking supplements.

Sources of omega-6

Omega-6 fats are important for brain development, too. They are found in seed oils such as sunflower and sesame. The more potent form of omega-6 fat is called gamma-linolenic acid (GLA). This is found in borage and evening primrose oil. The brain also needs arachidonic acid (AA), which can be made from GLA. It is found in the highest quantities in food of an animal origin such as fish, meat, eggs and dairy produce. We recommend supplementing some GLA along with omega-3 fish oils.

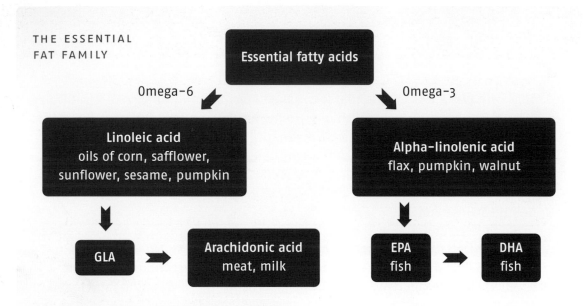

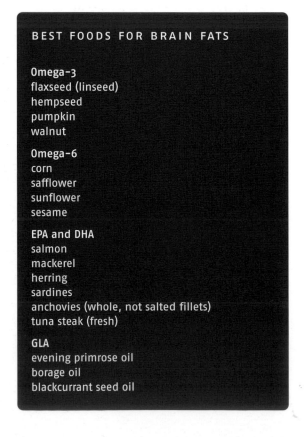

BEST FOODS FOR BRAIN FATS

Omega-3
flaxseed (linseed)
hempseed
pumpkin
walnut

Omega-6
corn
safflower
sunflower
sesame

EPA and DHA
salmon
mackerel
herring
sardines
anchovies (whole, not salted fillets)
tuna steak (fresh)

GLA
evening primrose oil
borage oil
blackcurrant seed oil

Which are the best fish to eat?

The best fish for omega-3s are carnivorous fish such as salmon and mackerel. The bigger the fish the more omega-3 it's likely to contain – marlin and swordfish are among the highest, followed by tuna. But we recommend tuna only once a week and marlin or swordfish no more than twice a month because these bigger fish are more likely to contain higher concentrations of mercury.

The seeds of life

Seeds are not only full of essential fats but they also contain lots of protein and vital minerals such as calcium, magnesium and

QUESTIONNAIRE: IS YOUR CHILD GETTING ENOUGH ESSENTIAL FATS?

Check whether your child is short on the healthy fats with the questionnaire below. Tick any of the boxes if your answer is 'yes'.

SYMPTOMS

Does your child have:

1 Dry or rough, bumpy skin or a tendency to have eczema? ☐

2 Brittle, dry or peeling nails? ☐

3 Dry or dull hair, or dandruff? ☐

4 Dry, watery or itchy eyes? ☐

5 Excessive thirst and/or frequent urination? ☐

6 Mood swings or tantrums? ☐

7 A poor memory, attention span or concentration? ☐

8 Poor physical coordination, or is clumsy? ☐

9 Slow or poor wound healing? ☐

10 Obsessive or compulsive behaviour? ☐

11 Phobia, extreme fears or night terrors? ☐

12 Anxiety or depression? ☐

13 Travel or motion sickness? ☐

14 Fits or convulsions? ☐

DIET

Does your child:

1 Eat oily fish such as salmon, mackerel, sardines or fresh tuna less than three times a week? ☐

2 Eat seeds, unroasted nuts (such as pumpkin, sunflower seeds or almonds), and/or unfried, cold-pressed seed oils on food or in salad dressings less than three times a week? ☐

3 Eat meat or dairy products most days? ☐

4 Often eat fried food, takeaway food or foods cooked in heated fat? ☐

5 Often eat processed foods (such as ready meals, chips or crisps)? ☐

6 Typically not take an essential-fat supplement? ☐

If you have ticked five or more of the boxes above, the chances are your child isn't getting enough essential fats. By upping your child's intake, these symptoms can rapidly improve.

zinc, as well as vitamin E. So eating some seeds every day is a smart move.

We recommend using seeds in three ways:

1   Adding ground seeds to food, whether it's cereals or soups (where they can be stirred in to make them invisible to beady-eyed, suspicious eaters). See the box opposite for the perfect seed mix.
2   Using cold-pressed seed oils for salad dressings and drizzled over hot food, such as vegetables, instead of butter.
3   Adding seeds to sauces, main meals and desserts. You must try our fabulous Chocolate or Banana Cheesecakes, for example, with finely chopped nuts and seeds in the biscuit base, or our Plum Crumble, which mixes ground almonds into an oaty topping.

Go to school on an egg

Eggs contain important brain fats called phospholipids. Phospholipids, also found in fish and organ meats, enhance your child's mood, mind and mental performance.

If you fry an egg the phospholipids, as well as the essential fats, will be damaged. So, it's better to have boiled, scrambled or poached egg than fried. See page 76 in the Breakfast section on for plenty of healthy egg-based recipes.

Eggs do contain cholesterol but there's no evidence that eating eggs promotes high blood-cholesterol levels or increases the risk of heart disease. That is a myth. But eggs are high in fat and the kind of fat depends on what the chicken eats. That's why we recommend you spend a little extra and buy organic or free-range eggs from chickens fed on flaxseeds (linseeds). These are described as omega-3-rich eggs and are available in supermarkets.

Avoid bad fats

When a food is deep fried, the frying not only destroys any goodness in the oil but also the high temperature damages essential fats in the food that is being fried. So, for example, it's better to have grilled or poached fish than to fry it. We'll show you how in the Healthy Cooking section on page 65.

Strictly avoid any processed foods that contain 'hydrogenated' fats, or trans-fats, found in foods such as doughnuts and ready meals. These are damaged fats and are no good for you.

Supplementing essential fats

As well as eating more fish and seeds, it's worth supplementing the essential fats every day. This way you guarantee your child is achieving optimum nutrition. This is especially important if your child is vegetarian, as the omega-3 fat (ALA) found in seeds such as flaxseed (linseed) isn't converted in your body into the critical brain-building fat, DHA, in any appreciable amounts. However, there are some supplements of DHA and EPA derived from seaweed becoming available for strict vegetarians.

The best supplements provide both EPA and DHA, as well as the omega-6 fat GLA. The following chart lists the daily levels of supplements we recommend you give your child:

Essential fat (mg):	Age: Less than 1	1	2	3–4	5–6	7–8	9–11	12–13
GLA	50	75	95	110	135	135	135	135
EPA	100	150	200	250	300	350	400	400
DHA	100	125	150	175	200	225	250	250

Choose supplements from a reputable company that guarantees they are pure and contain no mercury or PCBs, for example. Check that they contain all three essential fats (EPA, DHA and GLA), given in the amounts shown in the chart above (see Resources for recommendations).

 THE PERFECT SEED MIX

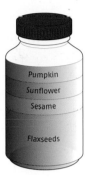

1. Take a glass jar with a sealing lid and half-fill with flaxseeds (linseeds), the only seed especially high in omega-3 fats. Fill the other half with mixed sesame, sunflower and pumpkin seeds. Shake to combine.
2. Keep the jar sealed, and in the fridge to minimise damage from light, heat and oxygen.
3. Put a mixed handful in a coffee grinder or nut mill, grind up and add to cereals or soups or, alternatively, munch a handful.
4. Children need two teaspoons a day, teenagers and adults need one tablespoon a day.

 GOLDEN RULE NO.1 — ENSURE ESSENTIAL FATS

* Eat oily fish two to three times a week.
* Eat seeds (especially flaxseeds (linseeds) and pumpkin seeds) daily.
* Eat three to six eggs (especially omega-3-rich eggs) a week.
* Supplement a capsule of EPA, DHA and GLA daily.
* Minimise deep-fried foods and foods containing hydrogenated and trans-fats.

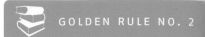
CHAPTER 3

Eat a Low-Sugar and Low-GL Diet

Ever picked your child up from a birthday party and opened the door on a roomful of kids bouncing off the walls? All that sugar has an amazingly dramatic effect on the brain. So it's hardly surprising that in daily life, too, overdoing the sweet stuff affects your child's behaviour.

Getting the right kind of sugar

Nothing is more important for your child's brain than sugar – blood sugar, or glucose, that is. It's the brain's main fuel, so without an adequate supply we can't think clearly. We get it from the carbohydrates in the foods we eat. The trick lies in keeping that supply even.

Too much, and you get the wall-bouncing effect. Too little, and your child could experience symptoms like fatigue, irritability, dizziness, insomnia, aggression, anxiety, sweating (especially at night), poor concentration, excessive thirst, depression, crying spells or blurred vision. So, for your child to be able to think with clarity and behave rationally, it's vital that their glucose supply stays steady and even.

So, what do you need to do to improve your child's blood sugar balance and banish these symptoms?

Eat low-GL foods

The measure of what a food does to your blood sugar is known as the Glycemic Load (GL). The sugars and starches in foods with a high GL (refined carbohydrates, such as white bread, sweets and biscuits) are broken down and absorbed quickly into the bloodstream making your child's blood glucose levels soar. Your child is likely to experience a sudden burst of energy followed by an energy crash. Meanwhile, the sugars and starches in foods with a low GL (complex carbohydrates such as whole grains, vegetables, beans or lentils, or with simpler carbohydrates such as fruit) take longer to digest than refined carbohydrates. As a result, the glucose released from these foods trickles slowly into the bloodstream. This means that it's used for energy rather than being stored, leaving blood glucose levels on an even keel, and preventing dramatic changes in mood, behaviour and energy.

QUESTIONNAIRE: IS YOUR CHILD GETTING TOO MUCH SUGAR?

Check whether your child is eating too much sugar with the questionnaire below. Tick any of the boxes if your answer is 'yes'.

SYMPTOMS

Does your child:

1 Seem slow to get going in the morning? ☐

2 Crave something sweet to eat or a cup of tea in the morning? ☐

3 Have difficulty sleeping or sleep restlessly? ☐

4 Have energy slumps during the day? ☐

5 Lack energy or complain of frequent tiredness? ☐

6 Lose concentration or have a poor attention span? ☐

7 Experience dizzy spells, suffer from brain fog or can't think straight? ☐

8 Become irritable, have mood swings and/or emotional outbursts or tantrums? ☐

9 Avoid physical exercise due to tiredness? ☐

10 Crave sweet foods/have a sweet tooth? ☐

DIET

Does your child:

1 Sometimes skip meals, especially breakfast? ☐

2 Eat refined foods – white rice, white bread, white pasta? ☐

3 Eat sugar, sweets or chocolate, biscuits, toast and jam or sweetened cereals? ☐

4 Often drink sugared drinks (such as colas, 'sports' drinks, sugared fruit drinks)? ☐

5 Often have cups of tea, coffee or cola (caffeinated) drinks? ☐

6 Often add teaspoons of sugar to drinks or cereals? ☐

If you have ticked five or more of the boxes above, the chances are your child's blood sugar balance is less than perfect.

The carbs that keep blood sugar even

The chart opposite gives the GL score of an average serving of a range of common foods. Foods with a GL of less than ten (highlighted in green) are good and should be the staple foods of your child's diet. A GL of 11 to 14 (highlighted in blue) can be eaten in moderation. A GL higher than 15 (highlighted in red) should be avoided. Fiona's recipes in Part 2 are low GL and help to balance blood sugar levels.

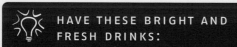

HAVE THESE BRIGHT AND FRESH DRINKS:

Water, fruity/herbal teas, diluted fruit juice (gradually increase the amount of water to let your child's taste buds adjust), diluted apple and blackcurrant concentrate such as Meridian, and fruit smoothies (a blend of fresh fruit and natural yoghurt, diluted with water, apple juice or milk).

GLYCEMIC LOAD OF COMMON FOODS

Food	Serving size in g	Looks like	GLs per serving
Bakery products			
low-carb muffin	–	1 muffin	5
muffin – apple, made without sugar	60	1 muffin	9
muffin – apple, made with sugar	60	1 muffin	13
crumpet	50	1 crumpet	13
croissant	57	1 croissant	17
doughnut	47	1 plain doughnut	17
sponge cake, plain	63	1 slice	17
Breads			
wholemeal rye or pumpernickel bread	20	1 thin slice	5
wheat tortilla (Mexican)	30	1 tortilla	5
wholemeal wheat flour bread	30	1 thick slice	9
pitta bread, white bread	30	1 pitta	10
baguette, white, plain	30	1/9 baton	15
bagel, white, frozen	70	1 bagel	25
Crispbreads and crackers			
rough oatcakes (Nairn's)	10	1 oatcake	2
fine oatcakes (Nairn's)	9	1 oatcake	3
cream cracker	25	2 biscuits	11
rye crispbread	25	2 biscuits	11
water cracker	25	3 biscuits	17
puffed rice cakes	25	3 biscuits	17
Dairy products and alternatives			
plain yoghurt (no sugar)	200	1 small pot	3
soya yoghurt (Provamel)	200	1 large bowl	7
soya milk (no sugar)	(250ml)	1 glass	7
low-fat yoghurt, fruit, sugar (Ski)	150	1 small pot	7.5
Breakfast cereals			
porridge made from rolled oats	30	1 small bowl	2
All-bran (Kellogg's)	30	1 small bowl	6

Food	Serving size in g	Looks like	GLs per serving
Muesli (Alpen)	30	1 small bowl	10
Weetabix	25	2 biscuits	11
Frosties (Kellogg's)	30	1 small bowl	15
Rice Crispies (Kellogg's)	30	1 small bowl	21
Cornflakes (Kellogg's)	30	1 small bowl	21
Fruit and fruit products			
blackberries, raw	120	1 medium bowl	1
raspberries, raw	120	1 medium bowl	1
strawberries, raw	120	1 medium bowl	1
pear, raw	120	1 medium	4
melon/cantaloupe, raw	120	½ small	4
watermelon, raw	120	1 medium slice	4
oranges, raw	120	1 large	5
plum, raw	120	4	5
apples, raw	120	1 small	6
kiwi fruit, raw	120	1	6
pineapple, raw	120	1 medium slice	7
grapes, raw	120	16	8
apricots, dried	60	6	9
banana, raw	120	1 small	12
sultanas	60	30	25
raisins	60	30	28
Vegetables			
broccoli	100	1 handful	2
carrots	80	1 small	3
green peas	80	1½ tbsp	3
boiled potato	150	3 small	14
baked potato, white baked in skin	150	1 large	18
french fries	150	20	22
Jams/spreads			
pumpkin seed butter	16	1 tbsp	1
peanut butter (no sugar)	16	1 tbsp	1
orange marmalade	10	2 teaspoons	3
strawberry jam	10	2 teaspoons	3

Food	Serving size in g	Looks like	GLs per serving
Snack foods (savoury)			
eggs (boiled)	–	2 medium	0
cottage cheese	120	½ medium tub	2
egg mayonnaise	120	½ medium tub	2
hummus	200	1 small tub	6
olives, in brine	50	7	1
peanuts	50	2 medium handfuls	1
cashew nuts, salted	50	2 medium handfuls	3
potato crisps, plain, salted	30	1 small packet	7
popcorn, salted	25	1 small packet	10
pretzels, oven-baked, traditional wheat flavour	30	15	16
corn chips, plain, salted	50	18	17
Snack foods (sweet)			
Fruitus apple cereal bar	35	1	5
Euroviva Rebar fruit and veg bar	50	1	8
muesli bar with dried fruit	30	1	13
chocolate bar, milk, plain (Mars/Cadbury/Nestlé)	50	1	14
Twix biscuit and caramel bar (Mars)	60	1 bar (2 fingers)	17
Snickers bar (Mars)	60	1	19
Jelly beans, assorted colours	30	9	22
Mars Bar	60	1	26
Complete dishes			
pasta with pesto	200	large plate	18
hamburger	120	medium	25
pizza (thick base)	300	large slice	36

(A comprehensive list of the GL value of foods is available in *The Holford Low-GL Diet*, or online at www.holforddiet.com.)

Eat carbohydrate with *fibre* and protein

The more fibre and protein you include with any meal or snack, the slower the release of the carbohydrates, which is good for blood–glucose balance. So, combining protein-rich foods with high-fibre carbohydrates is an excellent rule of thumb in this context. Here's how you do it:

* Eat seeds or nuts with a fruit snack.
* Add seeds or nuts to carbohydrate-based breakfast cereals.
* Top toast with eggs, baked beans or nut butter.
* Serve salmon or chicken with brown basmati rice – or try our delicious Egg Fried Rice recipe on page 107.
* Add kidney beans to pasta sauce served over wholemeal pasta.
* Put cottage cheese on oatcakes, or hummus on pumpernickel-style rye bread.
* Make sandwiches with sugar-free peanut butter and wholemeal bread.

Don't go without breakfast

Getting the kids up on a school morning with enough time for them to eat a decent breakfast can be challenging at the best of times. But eating a decent breakfast really is essential for your child to be able to concentrate at school. If their blood sugar level stays rock-bottom all morning, they'll experience all the problems we have mentioned, from dizziness to a lack of mental focus. If you struggle to get food down your child first thing in the morning, or have no time to sit them down in front of a bowl or plate of food, try our smoothie recipes for instant meals in a glass that can be drunk on the go (see Breakfasts, page 65).

We find that children who eat a nutritious diet generally get a much better night's sleep, too. The knock-on effect is that it's easier for them to get out of bed in the morning – which in turn gives them the time and inclination to eat a decent breakfast.

Stay off the caffeine

Sugar isn't the only factor in blood sugar problems. Stimulants are, too – and as caffeine is a powerful one, it can be highly disruptive to your child's blood sugar balance. The biggest culprits are cola and energy drinks, chocolate bars and chocolate drinks, tea and coffee. Instead you could try fruity herbal teas or rooibosch (redbush) tea if your child has already got into the habit of having hot drinks, or give them a fruit smoothie. They may experience 'withdrawal' symptoms, such as headaches, when they give up caffeine but these will disappear within a couple of days.

GOLDEN RULE NO. 2 – EAT A LOW-GL DIET

* Choose foods with a low GL and avoid foods with a high GL.
* Avoid overly processed foods and refined 'white' foods.
* Avoid sugar and foods containing sugar.
* Combine protein foods with carbohydrate foods.
* Make sure your child is eating fruit and vegetables every day.
* Choose real fresh fruit juices from the chill cabinet and dilute 50:50. Steer clear of the highly processed kind with a long shelf life.
* Encourage your child to eat breakfast.
* Help your child avoid caffeinated food and drinks, such as cola, tea and coffee.

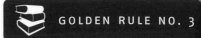

CHAPTER 4

Increase Vitamins and Minerals

In every great production, there are hundreds of people behind the scenes supporting the main players. The same is true of your child's brain – it's just that the heroes behind the lights, camera and action are vitamins and minerals, rather than technicians and casting agents.

Vitamins, minerals and IQ

One of the main roles of vitamins and minerals is to help turn glucose into energy, amino acids into neurotransmitters, simple essential fats into more complex fats like GLA or DHA, and choline and serine into phospholipids. They are key to the task of building and rebuilding the brain and nervous system, and keeping everything running smoothly. And they can help increase IQ, too. In the early 1980s we decided to test what would happen to the intelligence of schoolchildren if given an optimal intake of vitamins and minerals.[7] After eight months on the supplements, the non-verbal IQs in those taking the supplements had risen by nine points! Since then, ten out of 13 studies have shown IQ-boosting effects from giving children multivitamins.[8]

The B vitamins

B vitamins are absolutely key to mental health. The brain uses a huge amount of them and, as they're water-soluble and pass rapidly out of the body, even a short-term deficiency in any one of the eight Bs can result in a rapid shift in how your child thinks and feels. So it's best for them to get a regular intake throughout the day.

B deficiencies – the homocysteine link

How do you know if your child is getting enough B vitamins? One of the best gauges is homocysteine, a toxic protein found in the blood. If your child's level of blood homocysteine is high, they are likely to be low in B_6, B_{12} or folic acid because these vitamins help get rid of homocysteine. So they'll need to top up their Bs.

The ideal level of blood homocysteine for an adolescent or adult is below 7μmol/l. For a child of ten or younger, the level should ideally lie below 5μmol/l. See the Resources section (page 151) for details of how to get

QUESTIONNAIRE: IS YOUR CHILD GETTING ENOUGH VITAMINS AND MINERALS?

Check whether you need to increase your child's vitamins and minerals with the questionnaire below. Tick any of the boxes if your answer is 'yes'.

SYMPTOMS

Does your child:

1 Have poor night vision or hate bright lights? ☐

2 Have muscle cramps or spasms? ☐

3 Have white marks on more than two fingernails? ☐

4 Have poor appetite, or sense of taste or smell? ☐

5 Catch colds, flu, sore throats or infections? ☐

6 Have pale skin or spots/acne or bad skin? ☐

7 Bruise easily? ☐

8 Have mouth ulcers? ☐

9 Seem depressed or disconnected, avoid group activities or have difficulty relating with others? ☐

DIET

Does your child:

1 Eat fewer than five servings of fresh fruit and vegetables (excluding potato) every day? ☐

2 Eat less than one portion of a dark green vegetable a day? ☐

3 Eat fewer than three portions of fresh or dried tropical fruit a week? ☐

4 Eat seeds or seed oils (such as pumpkin, sunflower, tahini) or unroasted nuts less than three times a week? ☐

5 Usually eat white bread, rice or pasta instead of brown/wholegrain? ☐

6 Typically not take a multivitamin/mineral supplement? ☐

If you have ticked five or more of the boxes above, the chances are your child isn't getting enough vitamins and minerals.

your child tested. You might want to do this if your child is experiencing learning or behaviour problems. Alternatively, make sure that they take a multivitamin supplement containing optimal amounts of these B vitamins.

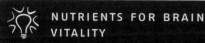

NUTRIENTS FOR BRAIN VITALITY

Every one of the 50 known essential vitamins and minerals plays a major role in promoting mental health. In the chart opposite we list the most vital to the condition of your child's brain, along with the symptoms you might see if your child is deficient, and the best food families to feed your child to ensure they get enough.

KEY VITAMINS AND MINERALS FOR SMART KIDS

Nutrient	Symptoms of deficiency	Food source
B₁	poor concentration and attention	wholegrains, vegetables
B₃	depression, psychosis	wholegrains, vegetables
B₄	poor memory, stress	wholegrains, vegetables
B₆	irritability, poor memory, depression, stress	wholegrains, bananas
folic acid	anxiety, depression, psychosis	green leafy vegetables
B₁₂	confusion, poor memory, psychosis	meat, fish, dairy products, eggs
vitamin C	depression, psychosis	vegetables, fresh fruit
magnesium	irritability, insomnia, depression, hyperactivity	green vegetables, nuts, seeds
manganese	dizziness, convulsions	nuts, seeds, tropical fruit
zinc	confusion, blank mind, depression, loss of appetite, lack of motivation and concentration	oysters, nuts, seeds, fish

Antioxidants – protecting your child's brain

We live in a highly polluted world, and there may not be a lot you can do to avoid many of the pollutants. But you can protect your child's brain from the inside, with antioxidants. Antioxidants are the antidote to oxidants, also known as 'free radicals' – highly unstable molecules that can trigger cellular damage. They are a by-product of the normal body processes and of combustion.

Combating oxidants

In the body, oxidants are produced every time glucose is 'burned' within a cell to make energy. In the environment, they are found in cigarette smoke, exhaust fumes and crispy, fried food. These have a harmful effect on your child's body and brain. To give your child maximum protection, it's worth making sure their daily supplement contains antioxidants, as well as giving them foods that are high in them, such as:

* **Beta-carotene** Carrots, sweet potatoes, dried apricots (soaked first), squash, watercress
* **Vitamin C** Broccoli, peppers, kiwi fruit, berries, tomatoes, citrus fruit
* **Vitamin E** Seeds and their cold-pressed oils, wheatgerm, nuts, beans, fish, avocados
* **Selenium** Oysters, brazil nuts, seeds, molasses, tuna, mushrooms
* **Glutathione** Tuna, pulses, nuts, seeds, garlic, onions
* **Anthocyanidins** Berries, cherries, red grapes, beetroot, prunes

Cooking healthily to avoid oxidants

Be aware that maximising your child's mental powers isn't just about what your child eats. It's also about what he or she *doesn't* eat. For example, eating a piece of crispy meat introduces millions of these oxidants. So it is important not to overcook, burn or char food. A barbecue is great fun, but do cook on lower flames and ensure your children's sausages are gently browned and cooked all the way through – not charred black on the outside. See Healthy Cooking on page 60.

Calcium and magnesium

These two minerals help to relax nerve and muscle cells. A lack of either calcium or magnesium can make children nervous, irritable and aggressive, yet magnesium is typically the second most commonly deficient mineral after zinc in children (muscle cramps are an obvious sign of magnesium deficiency). An ideal intake of magnesium is probably 300mg a day, which is almost double what most children achieve. But it's not hard to do: a tablespoon of seeds a day, two servings of a green vegetable, plus 30mg in a multimineral, is a good way to ensure your child is getting enough.

The best dietary sources of calcium, other than dairy products, are nuts (especially almonds), beans, lentils, seeds (especially sesame). If your child's diet is dairy-free make sure they are having the equivalent of a tablespoon of seeds (around 100mg), snacks of nuts or seeds (around 100mg), as well as eating beans or lentils (around 100mg), a calcium-enriched milk alternative (around 200–300mg), plus some extra calcium in their multivitamin supplement (40–200mg). In total you want them to achieve 500mg a day, or 800mg a day for teenagers. A cup of milk or yogurt provides around 300mg of calcium.

THE IDEAL DAILY SUPPLEMENT PROGRAMME

Age:	Less than 1	1–2	3–4	5–6	7–8	9–11	12–13
Essential vitamins							
A (retinol)	500mcg	650	800	1,000	1,500	2,000	2,500
D	1mcg	1.4	1.75	2.25	2.5	2.75	3.0
E	13mg	16	20	23	30	40	50
C	100mg	150	300	400	500	600	700
B_1 (thiamine)	5mg	6	8	12	16	20	24
B_2 (riboflavin)	5mg	6	8	12	16	20	24
B_3 (niacin)	7mg	12	16	18	20	22	24
B_5 (pantothenic acid)	10mg	15	20	25	30	35	40
B_6 (pyridoxine)	5mg	7	10	12	16	20	25
B_{12}	5mcg	6.5	8	9	10	10	10
folic acid	100mcg	120	140	160	180	200	220
biotin	30mcg	45	60	70	80	90	100
Essential minerals							
calcium	150mg	165	180	190	200	210	220
magnesium	50mg	65	80	90	100	110	120
iron	4mg	5.5	7	8	9	10	10
zinc	4mg	5.5	7	8	9	10	10
manganese	300mcg	350	400	500	700	1,000	1,000
iodine	40mcg	50	60	70	80	90	100
chromium	15mcg	19	23	25	27	30	30
selenium	10mcg	18	20	24	26	28	30
copper	400mcg	550	700	800	900	1,000	1,000
Essential fats							
GLA	50mg	75	95	110	135	135	135
EPA	100mg	175	250	300	350	350	350
DHA	100mg	140	175	200	225	225	225

Other brain nutrients (optional)

phosphatidyl choline	250–400mg
phosphatidyl serine	20–45mg
DMAE	200–300mg
glutamine	250–1,000mg
arginine pyroglutamate	300–450mg
trimethyl glycine (TMG)	250mg–1,000mg

Zinc

The most commonly deficient mineral, and one of the most critical nutrients for mental health, is zinc. This is particularly true for children since zinc is necessary for growth. A deficiency in this mineral is associated with hyperactivity, autism, depression, anxiety, anorexia, schizophrenia and delinquency – in short, it's implicated in a huge range of mental health problems. Sure signs of zinc deficiency are stretch marks, white spots on the fingernails and teenage acne. You'll find zinc in any 'seed' food – nuts, seeds and the germ of grains as well as meat and fish.

Supplements for Superkids

A varied and nutritious diet is the keystone of good health. But sometimes even the best diets fail to provide appropriate levels of all the nutrients we need, and some children need more of certain nutrients than others. Also, as we know, children can be picky eaters, so using supplements can be helpful.

Supplementation is the most reliable way to ensure your child gets all the vitamins and minerals they need to be optimally nourished. This is even more important if your child is having mental or emotional difficulties. A small deficiency in any one vitamin or mineral essential for good health could have a serious impact on your growing child.

Finding a good multi

There are many single multivitamin and mineral supplements available for children (see Resources). See the chart opposite for guidelines on the levels of nutrients to look for. You can choose chewable (or crushable in the early stages), or soluble formulas.

Ideally, give your child the supplement with breakfast, but not last thing at night, as the B vitamins can have a mild stimulatory effect (as can glutamine in some children). Children also tend to be more susceptible to vitamin toxicity than adults, so don't be tempted to give much more than these recommended, very safe levels unless under the direction and supervision of a nutritional therapist.

Alternatively, there are 'shake' powders that you can either add to cereal or whizz up with milk (or soya or rice milk) and fruit that are the equivalent of a multivitamin. Try 'Get Up & Go' (see Resources).

Essential fats to boost IQ

As long as your child is eating oily fish three times a week and a daily portion of seeds (see page 23), they should be getting sufficient essential fats. However, if they don't eat fish or don't have seeds every day, we recommend you supplement their diet with an essential fat formula. Look for one that contains GLA (omega-6), DHA and EPA, and use the chart as a guide to quantities. The most important essential fat is omega-3 and there are many different forms of supplements available, ranging from pastes to drinks to tiny capsules. You can always pierce a capsule and add it to juice or food.

Extra brain nutrients

There are also 'brain food' nutrients that are worth supplementing if you find your child is struggling. Look for a specific 'brain food' formula that contains phospholipids (phosphatidyl choline, serine and DMAE), glutamine and pyroglutamate. However, they usually come in tablets that might be hard for a younger child to swallow. For phosphatidyl choline (PC) you can add some lecithin granules to cereal, giving two teaspoonfuls of regular lecithin or one teaspoonful of hi-PC lecithin. Glutamine comes in a powder that easily dissolves in water or diluted juice.

The chart on page 34 shows the ideal daily amounts of vitamins, minerals and essential fats to supplement from weaning to age 13, combined with a reasonably healthy diet. Once a child is 14, adult amounts of nutrients apply. You can find these in Chapter 45 of *Patrick Holford's New Optimum Nutrition Bible* or at www.patrickholford.com/supplements.

 GOLDEN RULE NO. 3 — INCREASE VITAMINS AND MINERALS

* Make sure your child eats plenty of foods rich in antioxidants — fruits, vegetables, seeds and fish.
* Serve nuts and seeds daily.
* Choose wholefoods (those that have had little added or taken away).
* Choose wholegrains (wholemeal bread, oats, brown rice, wholemeal pasta).
* Don't smoke, and keep your kids away from smoky places. Don't overcook, deep fry or chargrill food.
* Make sure your child takes an 'optimum nutrition' multivitamin/mineral every day.

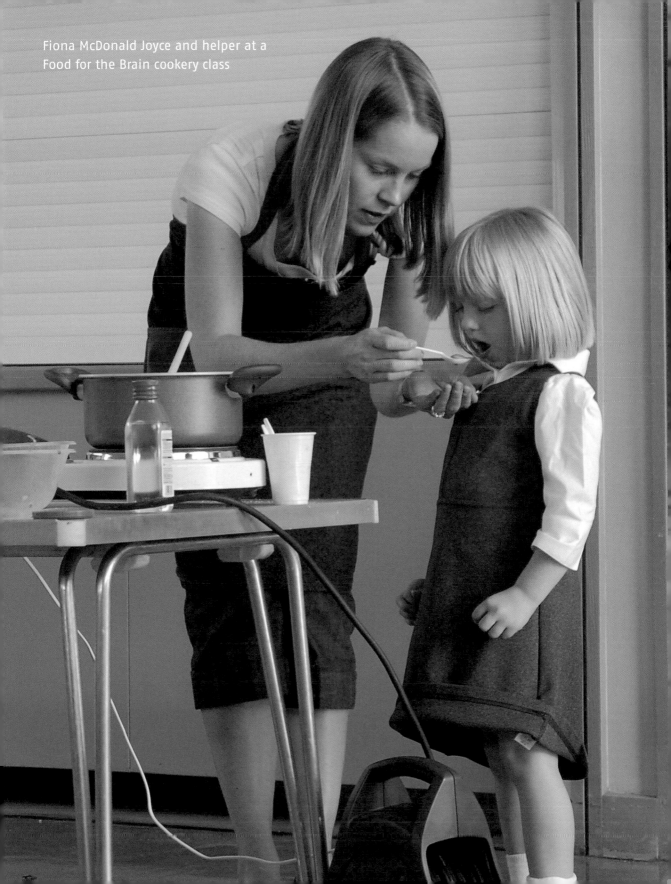

Fiona McDonald Joyce and helper at a
Food for the Brain cookery class

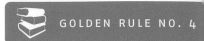

CHAPTER 5

Consider Food Allergies and Chemical Sensitivities

As many as one in five adults and children,[9,10] and probably one in three children with behavioural problems, have allergic reactions to foods such as milk, wheat, yeast and eggs. Although it has been known for a long time that allergies to foods and chemicals can adversely affect moods and behaviour in children, this knowledge has largely been ignored.

Yet allergies can cause a diverse range of symptoms, including fatigue, slowed thought processes, irritability, agitation, aggressive behaviour, nervousness, anxiety, depression, ADHD, autism, hyperactivity and learning disabilities[11–18].

Understanding the differences

People often use the terms 'food allergies', 'food intolerances' and 'food sensitivities' almost interchangeably. So, what is the difference between them? The classic definition of an allergy is simply an exaggerated physical reaction to a substance involving the immune system. This can be an immediate and severe reaction to a food – such as peanuts – that may be life-threatening. If your child has this type of allergy, you probably already know about it and are strictly keeping your child away from the offending food. But the most common food allergies can take from one hour to 24 hours to emerge and are often less immediately dramatic and harder to detect – such as allergies to wheat and dairy. So it's more likely your child will continue to eat these foods.

Food intolerances and sensitivities

An intolerance or sensitivity is a reaction to a food where there is no measurable antibody response. Examples include lactose intolerance, where a child lacks the enzyme to digest lactose (milk sugar), usually resulting in digestive symptoms such as diarrhoea and tummy pains, or intolerance to the flavour enhancer MSG (monosodium glutamate), which makes some kids hyperactive.

Testing for allergies

If you suspect your child might have an allergy, you can arrange for an allergy test. The best test, called IgG ELISA, uses a finger-prick blood sample and is available as a home-test kit (see Resources). Testing is best done under the guidance of a nutritional therapist or allergy expert who can then devise a suitable diet.

QUESTIONNAIRE: IS YOUR CHILD ALLERGIC?

Check whether your child has an allergy by taking the questionnaire below. Tick any of the boxes if your answer is 'yes'.

SYMPTOMS

Does your child:

1 Have asthma? ☐

2 Have eczema, skin rashes, itches or dermatitis? ☐

3 Have a chronic stuffy or runny nose or catarrh? ☐

4 Repeatedly touch, pick or rub their nose? ☐

5 Have allergies, including hayfever? ☐

6 Have earaches/frequent ear infections? ☐

7 Have tonsillitis? ☐

8 Have dark circles under the eyes or puffy eyes? ☐

9 Have migraines or headaches? ☐

10 Have tummy aches, bloating, flatulence or diarrhoea? ☐

11 Crave certain foods (not sugar), such as milk or bread? ☐

12 React to, avoid or omit certain foods due to an intolerance or sensitivity? ☐

13 React to mould, dust, pets, chemicals, additives? ☐

DIET

Does your child:

1 Frequently eat wheat-based foods such as bread, rolls, pasta, biscuits, cakes, pastries or wheat cereal? ☐

2 Frequently eat dairy produce such as milk, cheese or yogurt? ☐

If you have ticked five or more of the boxes above, the chances are your child may have a food allergy, intolerance or sensitivity.

Alternatively, you can try an elimination-and-challenge diet. This involves removing any likely culprits from your child's diet for a month and noting any changes in behaviour, or mental and physical symptoms. Then the foods are reintroduced in a controlled way, and your child is monitored closely for any changes. This method has many shortcomings because the range of foods that a child can react to is so broad. If you are reducing dairy products (milk, cheese, yoghurt) your child will need an alternative source of calcium, such as a daily tablespoonful of seeds.

Keep your child chemical-free

A high intake of chemical additives in food has been associated with mood swings and aggressive behaviour, poor attention span, depression and apathy, disturbed sleep patterns, impaired memory and intellectual performance. The most commonly reported culprits are aspartame, tartrazine and MSG. It is best to avoid foods with chemical additives.

Go for organic

The presence of pesticide residues, particularly on fruits and vegetables, is widely acknowledged. Any toxic substance will affect all parts of the body, including the brain to some extent, so it seems wise to try to avoid pesticides and go for organic whenever you can.

GOLDEN RULE NO. 4 – CONSIDER FOOD ALLERGIES AND CHEMICAL SENSITIVITIES

* If your child scores high on allergic symptoms, take wheat and dairy products out of their diet completely for one month and see how they feel.
* If you suspect your child has a food allergy, have an IgG ELISA food allergy test and see a clinical nutritional therapist.
* Improve your child's digestion by including plenty of fresh fruit, vegetables and seeds in their diet.
* Keep antibiotics and painkillers to a minimum – they damage the digestive tract.
* Avoid foods containing chemical food additives.
* Stick to whole, natural foods as much as possible and check labels.
* Choose organic food whenever possible.

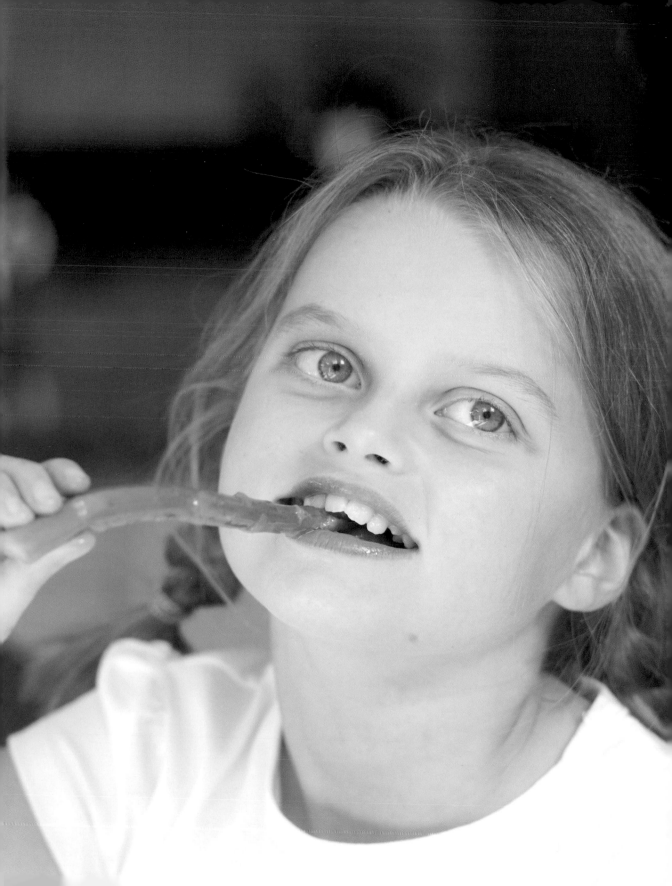

Part 2
by Fiona McDonald Joyce

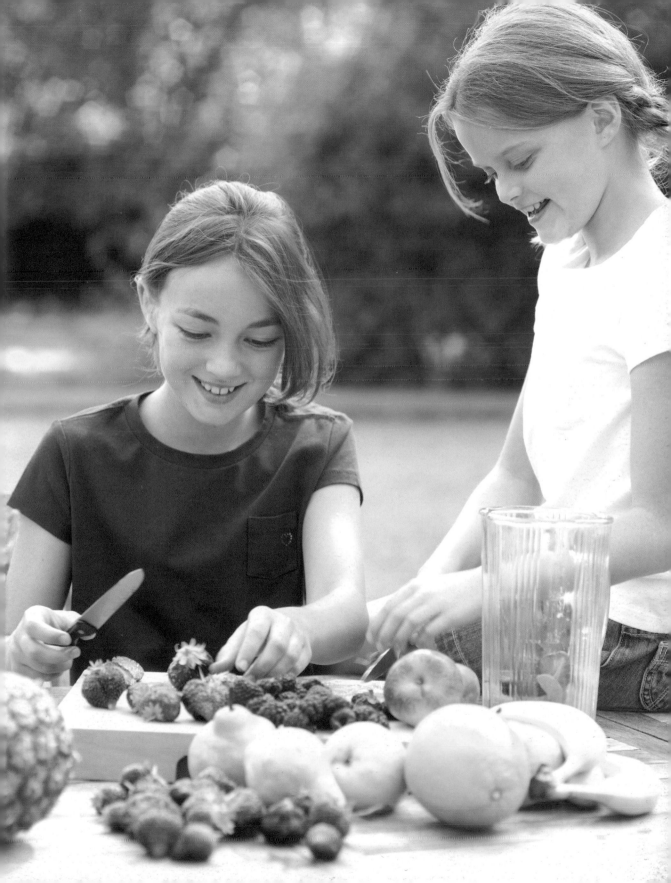

INTRODUCTION

Now for the fun – and messy – part: the cooking. These recipes are designed with three things in mind:

1. **To be quick and easy for parents short on time and energy,** and to encourage children to get involved in cooking (to this end we have highlighted which recipes are particularly suitable for children to make).
2. **To be suitable for all the family to enjoy,** to save separate cooking and to allow you to eat together as a family. The book is aimed at all children over five years, but is also suitable for teenagers and parents, as well as younger toddlers (see the Start Early note on page 48). We have made main meals to feed four, to suit most families, but you can easily halve the quantities, or double up to batch cook and freeze leftovers in order to save time.
3. **To be as delicious as they are nutritious,** to avoid mealtime battles and to show your child that healthy eating can taste great.

Tips for picky eaters, variations and serving suggestions are provided with recipes where appropriate. We have also highlighted those dishes that are rich in brain-boosting essential fatty acids (with the symbol ◗) and those suitable for vegetarians (with the symbol ⓥ) and for people on special diets, giving comprehensive details of the allergy suitability of each dish. Where possible, we have included alternatives for common allergens such as wheat and dairy products, and the allergy rating in the cook's notes of each recipe reflects this (for example, where we suggest using milk or a non-dairy milk, the allergy suitability will be listed as 'dairy-free').

Food that's fun as well as healthy

So often, books aimed at improving your child's diet fail to give them the food they will really like, and it is as important to us as it is to you that this book isn't the same. For this reason we have tried and tested all our recipes on lots of families, including our first Food for the Brain schools, giving them to parents to cook for their children at home.

Dishes have been given their seal of approval for speed, simplicity and success, passing their children's (and sometimes spouses') stringent taste tests! In fact, one father, John, described by his wife Marion as 'incredibly hard to please', was so taken with the new recipes that he asked: 'When we have finished all this recipe testing we aren't going back to the old food, are we?' Praise indeed! The result is a collection of recipes that should appeal to all tastes.

If you struggle with a picky eater, don't

despair, it takes time to change habits, and many children are incredibly suspicious about new foods, as well as seeing mealtimes as a means to exert some control. Start off slowly, by swapping some of their regular meals for the recipes here. You can monitor any improvements in your child's behaviour, mental performance and overall well-being using the chart on pages 148–9.

A note on fibre

Many of the ingredients featured in these recipes are high in dietary fibre, as these foods are packed with the vital vitamins and minerals required for physical and mental development. Younger children (especially the under twos) need less fibre, however, as it is so filling that their small tummies fill up rapidly, leaving no space for other valuable nutrients required for growth. If you are feeding younger children then make sure they are not filling up on high-fibre foods such as fruit, vegetables or wholegrains exclusively – they should still be eating protein and fat. Give them smaller servings of high-fibre foods so that they have room for these other foods, but at the same time get them used to eating healthy ingredients like wholemeal bread, fruit and vegetables.

Children used to a very low-fibre diet (featuring white bread and pasta, cakes and biscuits, and minimal fruit and vegetables) may also find that they get a runny tummy when switching to a high-fibre diet. For this reason, we suggest you make changes slowly.

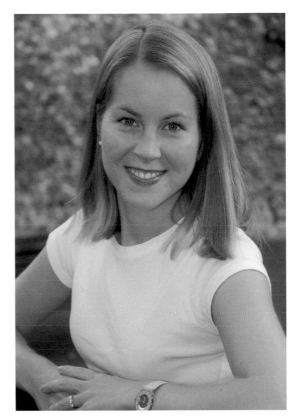

Fiona McDonald Joyce

So don't go from eating no fruit to five pieces per day, for example. Their digestive systems may need a little time to adjust to these new, nutritious foods if they are used to very low-fibre, nutrient-devoid processed food.

Everything in moderation

The other point worth raising is that we are not expecting your child to give up all their favourite drinks and foods. Food is not only meant to nourish us but it is also a chief pleasure in life, and the recipes in this book reflect this. However, unless you or your child are following a very restrictive diet for allergy or other health reasons, the 80:20 rule is a great rule to bear in mind: stick to the foods we recommend 80 per cent of the time, and you and your child can enjoy the occasional treat with a clean conscience. This also helps your child to develop a balanced, healthy attitude towards food so that they are not rushing to the nearest sweet shop whenever you are out of sight.

Here are some tips that parents of the pickiest of eaters at our Food for the Brain schools found particularly helpful:

Let them play with their food (up to a point!)

Bring out chopsticks one day; blindfold them for a 'guess what's for supper' food-tasting test another time; make them eat the different foods on their plate in alphabetical order – there are all kinds of games you can play to encourage your child to eat and to deflect attention from battles over whether they like a food or not.

Tiny titbits

Cut up food into small, bite-sized chunks, or even smaller, to make meals seem more manageable.

Bribery and corruption

Heap lots of praise and encouragement on your child when they eat healthy foods, and use incentives such as stickers, star charts or points. Make sure that you don't undo all your good work by making the treat one of the unhealthy items you have been weaning your child off; a treat doesn't have to be forbidden food or drink, but can be an extra-long bedtime story, a toy or a trip somewhere exciting. These reward schemes work particularly well when you have more than one child taking part; it's amazing what you can get children to do once you introduce a bit of healthy competition. If your child doesn't have any brothers or sisters, either get their friends' parents on board or speak to their teacher to introduce a 'Healthy Start Star Chart' at school.

Go shopping

Make food shopping fun, and get your child involved in more than just the sweet selection, by getting them to help you choose healthy foods. For example, get them to choose a new fruit, or select the greenest apple, or choose vegetables for a stir-fry.

Get cooking

At the Food for the Brain schools we saw so many children who claimed to hate all vegetables, but when we got them making Big Baked Beans (see page 111), which features tomatoes and onions, they wolfed them down. Likewise, most children will be happy to eat a stir-fry that they have helped to make.

Smart snacking

Snacks in between meals are a good idea to help keep blood sugar balanced so that your child's energy, concentration levels and mood remain stable, but you don't want your child to be so full of snacks that they don't eat at mealtimes. A mid-morning and mid-afternoon snack will keep most children filled up between meals, although very big or active children can have more, and if your child is used to constantly grazing, you can give them several 'mini meals' throughout the day, instead of three main meals and only a couple of snacks. The quantity of snacks is not as important as quality, however. Make sure that between-meal nibbles are nutritious, and low in sugar (see the Snacks section on page 78 to give you plenty of ideas).

Watch out for drinks, too – most juice drinks, squashes, fizzy drinks and flavoured milks contain as much sugar as many confectionery items, and milk is a protein and fat-rich food that will fill them up quickly so that they don't want meals.

Set a good example

Research conducted by Cancer Research UK has shown that while a taste for meat is inherited, a sweet tooth and a liking for vegetables is influenced by parents' food choices. They found that children were more likely to develop a taste for vegetables such as broccoli or carrots if their parents liked them, too, and the same goes for sweet puddings and snacks – suggesting that parents may have far more control over their children's diet than was first thought. Some Food for the Brain parents wouldn't even try the food samples we made at our parents' cookery sessions, so goodness knows how

they expected to persuade their children to eat them at home.

The best way to get your child to expand their diet is to eat together as a family, around the table, without the distractions of television, and to set a good example by eating the same foods that you expect them to eat yourself. Choose vegetables that you love and show them that you are enjoying your food.

Don't give up

Children's palates change as their taste buds develop, so if your child turns their nose up at peas, persevere, as research shows that it takes an average of ten 'tastes' for a child to accept a new food. Children will get used to anything – but if their taste buds get used to the high levels of salt, sugar and artificial flavourings that are in processed foods, of course they are going to find natural foods bland in comparison.

Attitude shift

It is worth considering how you treat food in your household:

* Is it really a treat for a child to be given a sugary or additive-ridden snack or drink that sends their behaviour out of control, so that they get into trouble?
* If you give your child a chocolate bar or fizzy drink every day then it is expected and no longer a treat.
* Don't give foods a 'good' or 'bad'

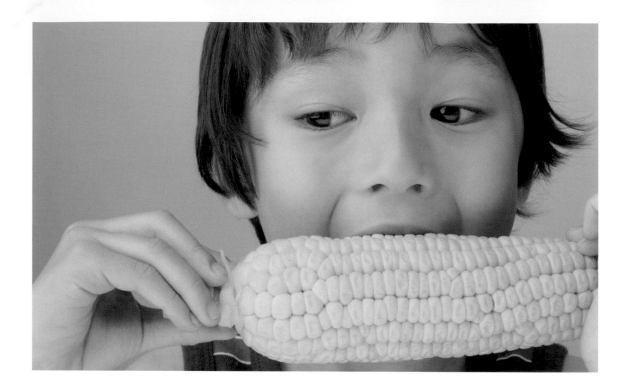

personality, as this can lead to disordered eating patterns in adulthood.

* Consider your own relationship with food – are you always on a diet, or do you binge on chocolate when you are bored or depressed? Children notice and absorb a lot of our own traits and habits.

Start early

It is much easier to prevent a poor diet than to remedy one. Once your child has got a taste for highly processed, sugary, salty and fatty foods, they will be loath to give them up. On this note, although the book is aimed at children over five years old, if you have younger toddlers the advice and recipes here still apply, and will help get them on the right track from the outset and develop a taste for

healthy foods. Children over the age of one should be eating more or less the same food and following the same meal patterns as the rest of the family, so they, too, should have three meals with two snacks in between. Obviously their taste buds will not be as developed as older children's, so you may wish to steer clear of some of the more adventurous ingredients such as chilli, and they won't need as much food, so as a rule of thumb, halve the portion size of the main meals to feed the under fives.

You will also need to limit their fibre intake, as their small tummies will fill up too quickly on bulky, high-fibre foods and they won't have space for other nutrients required for growth. Brown rice and pasta, wholemeal bread, oats, fruit and vegetables are all high in fibre, so manage your child's intake so that they don't fill up on these exclusively.

YOUR SHOPPING LIST

Use the following lists of healthy foods to stock up on all you need. A good supermarket will carry almost all the items that are listed here. You may find that a few are kept in the 'speciality foods' section or the 'healthy eating' aisle; alternatively, try your local health-food store.

There are also a number of web-based or mail-order companies that can deliver some of the healthy ingredients which are more difficult to source (see Resources for details). We have specified those items that should ideally be organic or free range, but this obviously depends very much on your budget and their availability. For more information see the Organic or Not? section on page 57.

Fresh fruits and vegetables

* **Plenty of fresh fruit**, in a rainbow of colours to maximise your child's intake of phyto (plant) nutrients. Choose fruits that are low GL, such as apples, pears, plums, apricots, berries, peaches, oranges and nectarines, in preference, and eat high-GL fruits (which are high in fruit sugars) in moderation, such as bananas, grapes, pineapples, mangoes, lychees and other tropical fruit. If you can, buy organic, particularly for those fruits that don't need peeling.

* **Bags of frozen mixed berries** These antioxidant-rich fruits are available in supermarkets and are an excellent way to include berries in your child's diet during the winter months. See the Winter Berry Smoothie (page 75) and the Instant Frozen Yogurt (page 126).

* **Plenty of fresh vegetables** Go for a range of different colours to ensure an intake of all the phyto-nutrient groups. Don't just go for starchy vegetables like potatoes and carrots – their starch is quickly converted to sugar so they will still raise the blood sugar level. Eat these in moderation, and, instead, your family can gorge on lettuce and salad leaves, cherry tomatoes, cucumber, courgette, broccoli, cauliflower, baby corn, peas, sugar snap peas and mangetouts, onions, peppers and beansprouts. Buy organic if possible, particularly for those vegetables that don't need peeling.

* **Sweet potatoes** are a real immune-system booster, and as they are naturally sweet and creamy you don't need to add extra butter or milk when mashing or baking them.

* **Organic baby new potatoes** As they are younger than larger types of potato, less of their starch has turned to sugar, so they won't upset blood sugar levels as much as larger potatoes.

* **Garlic** A good way to add flavour to dishes instead of salt, and a real superfood to boost the immune system and fight allergies.

* **Fresh root ginger** Another brilliant way to flavour food and add antioxidant power to keep your child fighting fit.

* **Lemons** Use unwaxed, if possible, for dressings and making homemade lemonade (see page 143).

* **Fresh herb growing pots** Much cheaper than sachets of pre-cut herbs, growing herbs in pots will give you a ready supply. Put your child in charge of looking after them (basil, flat-leaf parsley, coriander and chives are all easily available) to get them involved in food.

* **Sprouted seeds** such as cress or alfalfa sprouts. These are delicious in sandwiches and salads, and your child will enjoy growing them.

Foods for your fridge and freezer

* **Organic, semi-skimmed milk** or a dairy-free alternative such as soya, almond or hazelnut, or quinoa 'milk'. (Note that all these contain protein, helping to balance blood sugar, whereas rice milk is very high in starchy carbohydrates and has a high GL, so limit or avoid it if your child has blood sugar problems.)

GROWING AND SPROUTING SEEDS

Cress can easily be grown by sprinkling the seeds over pads of moistened cotton wool and watering regularly.

To sprout alfalfa seeds without a bean sprouter, soak 1 tbsp/15 ml seeds in water overnight. Put them into a clean glass jar and cover the top with muslin secured with a rubber band. Put in a warm, dark place. Twice a day pour water through the muslin and then carefully invert the jar to drain thoroughly. The sprouts will usually take about three days before they are ready to eat. They can be stored in the fridge.

* **Organic or free range eggs** are preferable from the point of view of taste, the welfare of the chickens and your own health. Eggs can be an excellent source of B vitamins, zinc, iron and phospholipids (fats required for cell membranes and a healthy brain), but they are only as good as the food the chicken was fed on. Look out for eggs from chickens fed on flaxseeds (linseeds), as these are a good source of omega-3 oils.

* **Low-fat cottage cheese and cream cheese** Organic brands are hard to find, but if you do see them, choose those.

* **Organic feta cheese** and soft, mild goat's cheeses.

* **Organic butter** A stable fat to cook with that is also free from the harmful

hydrogenated fats added to many margarines.

* **Organic live, natural yoghurt** Live sheep's or goat's yoghurt is more easily digested than cow's yoghurt.

* **Free range (or organic) chicken or turkey** (whole birds, breasts, thighs or drumsticks).

* **Organic salmon fillets** Salmon is usually better liked than other oily fish such as trout, mackerel, anchovies, sardines, herring, kippers and fresh tuna. Fresh tuna is a great source of omega-3 fats but as it accumulates heavy metals from polluted waters, it has been shown to contain high levels of mercury. Don't eat it more than once a month.

* **Smoked and unsmoked haddock fillets** (undyed), or other firm-fleshed white fish such as pollack.

* **Organic mince** Beef, lamb and turkey mince are all suitable.

* **Sausages** with a high lean-meat content, from good-quality butchers or farmers' markets.

* **Lean slices of ham on the bone** for sandwiches, salads and snacking.

* **Hummus** for sandwiches and snacks.

* **Bags of prepared frozen vegetables** such as broccoli florets, diced peppers and peas – for when you don't have time to prepare fresh.

* **Unsalted, unroasted nuts and seeds** for snacking and cooking. Although these won't be stored in the chill cabinet they should ideally be kept in your fridge to prevent their oils from oxidising and going rancid (you will know if they have gone off as they will taste bitter and revolting). Sunflower, pumpkin, sesame seeds and flaxseeds (linseeds) provide a good balance of omega-3 and omega-6 fats to sprinkle on cereals. Hazelnuts, walnuts, brazil nuts, pecan nuts and almonds are rich in minerals and essential fats but low in saturated fat (and ground almonds are very useful for baking). Peanuts, cashew nuts and macadamia nuts are fairly high in saturated fat, so limit these. Some people are allergic to nuts; seeds are much less allergenic, and flaxseeds (linseeds) and pumpkin seeds are particularly well tolerated. (See The Perfect Seed Mix on page 23.)

Store-cupboard staples

* **Dried or canned legumes and pulses** (peas, beans and lentils). Red lentils cook down to a soft porridge consistency, which is great in stews, soups, curries and Bolognese; Puy lentils, however, keep their shape when cooked. Chickpeas and beans such as borlotti, butter, kidney and flageolet, as well as canned mixed pulses, are all useful. If you go for canned, choose the ones canned in water, or drain and rinse thoroughly before use to remove as much salt and sugar as possible.

* **Baked beans** Popular with children and a good way to get them to eat pulses.

* **Canned tuna fish** A convenient store-cupboard stand-by, but don't rely on it too often, as tuna does accumulate any heavy metals from polluted waters it lives in.

* **Organic wholemeal bread or rye bread** (pumpernickel-style or sourdough), or an 'all-in-one' white bread 'with added goodness', which is very popular with children who refuse to eat wholemeal. Anyone avoiding wheat should check the labels carefully, as some rye breads include wheat. Most children find the flavour of pumpernickel-style rye bread too strong and the texture quite hard and chewy, but it is a useful alternative if your child is avoiding wheat and you can get them to eat it. It is more popular with older children.

* **Organic rough oatcakes** such as Nairn's are a good wheat-free alternative to bread and crackers. Rough oatcakes have a lower GL than finely milled varieties.

* **Organic wholemeal pasta** Choose a gluten-free variety such as brown rice or buckwheat pasta, if necessary; buckwheat has a lower GL than rice or corn pasta.

* **Organic brown basmati rice** The lowest GL of all rices, so it is more filling and less fattening. It has a nutty flavour and chewy texture and is far more interesting than plain white rice.

* **Organic soba noodles** Made from gluten-free buckwheat, these noodles cook very quickly and can be used hot or cold in salads and steam-fries or stir-fries. Look out for the 100 per cent buckwheat noodles sold in supermarkets, as some brands also contain wheat.

* **Quinoa** A South American fruit seed, pronounced 'keenwaa', which looks and cooks like a grain and is very similar to couscous. It contains all the essential amino acids, making it a perfect protein food, and it's also low in fat and rich in minerals.

* **Polenta flour or cornmeal** for gluten-free batters and coating Chicken Nuggets on page 98 and Fish Fingers on page 101.

* **Organic whole oats** Use for baking and cereals (see Breakfasts on page 65).

* **Coconut oil** The most stable oil for cooking. It's virtually flavourless and can be used for spreading, frying and baking – it is solid at room temperature and melts to an oil when heated. It will not raise cholesterol or produce harmful trans-fats when cooked, unlike polyunsaturated fats (see the Foods to Avoid section opposite). If you have difficulty obtaining coconut oil you can buy it from Health Products for Life (see the Company Directory on page 155).

* **Extra virgin olive oil** for salad dressings.

* **Sesame oil** for oriental dressings and dishes, and to enliven couscous, quinoa or rice salads.

* **Tamari** A wheat-free soy sauce that has a good, strong flavour.

* **Tahini** (ground sesame-seed paste). Useful as a spread and for making hummus.

* **Pesto** A sauce made with basil, pine nuts and Parmesan cheese, which can transform a simple pasta dish.

* **Canned coconut milk** A delicious alternative to creamy or tomato-based curried sauces.

* **Canned chopped tomatoes, tomato purée and sun-dried tomato paste** are all useful bases for sauces such as chilli, Bolognese and curries. Cooked tomatoes contain more of the antioxidant lycopene than raw ones, making these a really healthy addition to meals.

* **Olives** Avoid those that list colourings and additives on the label. Greek Kalamata olives are wonderfully moist and full of flavour. Buy ready-pitted to avoid children choking on the stones.

* **Nut butter** Choose sugar-free ones, and look in health-food stores for different types of nut and seed butter; there are cashew, sunflower, hazelnut and almond butters, as well as peanut butter.

* **Xylitol** A naturally sweet, low-carb sugar alternative (found in some plants) that doesn't disrupt blood sugar levels and has a third of the calories of sugar. Available in supermarkets and health-food stores (see Resources section on page 151). When first using xylitol, increase daily intake gradually to allow the body to adjust, as large quantities can have a laxative effect.

* **Good-quality chocolate** (about 50–70 per cent cocoa solids). Lower in sugar than cheap milk chocolate, which relies on added sugar to make up for the lack of cocoa solids. Good-quality chocolate contains iron and magnesium.

* **Black peppercorns** A good way to add flavour instead of salt. Plus, freshly ground black pepper contains a substance that helps you absorb nutrients.

* **Sea salt** To be used in moderation.

* **Marigold Reduced Salt Vegetable Bouillon powder** A delicious, full-flavoured alternative to stock cubes, it is suitable for vegans and is gluten-, yeast- and soya-free. It can also be added to dishes at any stage of cooking; there is no need to dissolve it in water like stock cubes. Most supermarkets stock it.

* **Dried herbs and spices** (such as herbes de Provence, mixed Italian herbs, oregano, chilli powder and chilli flakes, cayenne pepper, curry powder, ground cumin, coriander and turmeric).

Foods to avoid

* **Sunflower oil and vegetable oil for cooking** Although previously recommended as healthy options because they are low in saturated fat, in fact their lack of saturates makes them unstable at high temperatures, so they are damaged when heated and produce harmful trans-fats. Instead, use coconut oil (see opposite), butter or olive oil – but don't choose virgin olive oil for cooking as it has a low smoke point, and so gets damaged at high temperatures, and the taste that makes it so desirable is ruined upon heating, making it a waste of money.

* **Hydrogenated fats**, partially hydrogenated fats and trans-fats, found in margarines, many biscuits and cakes, and processed food. These man-made fats take up the positions of essential brain fats to disturb the thinking process.

* **Most E numbers**. Use our Green-Light E-Number Guide (on page 59) to check out the E numbers listed on processed foods.

* **White bread, pasta, rice and flour** White grains, breads and flours are devoid of the minerals, vitamins and fibre that are found in the wholegrains and wholemeal bread and flour.

* **'Brown' bread** Unless it says 'wholemeal' on the wrapper, brown bread is likely to be just white bread that has been coloured brown.

* **Cereals** Most of these are very high in sugar and additives, so read the labels carefully, and don't believe the marketing hype that these are healthy products. Work out the sugar content for yourself by using our guide on page 58. Beware of shop-bought mueslis and granolas, as these not only contain sugar but often also contain syrups, sweetened dried fruit and skimmed milk powder – all ways of adding extra sweetness on the sly. Health-food stores and some supermarkets do stock mueslis with no added salt or sugar, but the dried fruit still makes them quite high in fruit sugars. Choose wholegrain cereals and serve with chopped fresh fruit or xylitol to add natural sweetness.

* **Non-organic fizzy drinks** contain phosphoric acid, which the body neutralises by leaching calcium from the bones, thereby increasing the risk of developing osteoporosis in later years.

* **Sugar** See our list of all the different forms that sugar can take, on page 58. Sugar upsets blood sugar balance to cause weight gain and affect concentration and energy levels, as well as suppressing the immune system and rotting the teeth. Use xylitol instead (see Resources on page 153).

* **Artificial sweeteners** These may be low-calorie but some have been associated with worrying health concerns, including carbohydrate cravings. We recommend you sweeten foods with xylitol, a type of sugar found in some plants, which doesn't upset blood sugar balance (see page 153).

* **Battery-farmed eggs** Not only does buying battery-farmed eggs condone the appalling conditions in which the hens live, but the quality of the feed given to the hens is so poor that the nutritional quality of the egg suffers as a result.

* **Reconstituted meat** Cheap ham, luncheon meat, sausages, chicken nuggets, burgers and ready meals make use of the leftover parts of an animal that no one would touch with a bargepole if they could see them displayed in the butchers, including fat, skin and gristle. They are chemically bound back together and heavily disguised with additives, fillers and flavourings.

* **Non-organic soya products** There are a number of soya alternatives to sausages, burgers and other meats available, and many undergo harmful chemical processing and are heavily laced with flavourings to make them appear meaty and delicious. You would be far better off feeding your child a good-quality meat sausage or burger instead – at least you will know what it is that they are eating. Also, soya is the most genetically modified of all foods, so choose organic to minimise the risk. In fact, soya in general should be limited, as it is one of the most common allergens, and it also contains high amounts of phyto, or plant, oestrogens that can upset the delicate balance of your child's developing hormone system, as well as being goitrogenic (blocking the absorption of iodine and thereby upsetting thyroid function). So if your child doesn't have dairy products, don't use soya milk every day, for example – rotate it with other non-dairy milks like rice or almond milk, and don't give them tofu or other soya products (such as soya sausages or burgers) more than once a week.

* **Vegetarian mycoprotein products** Again, these are highly processed and flavoured and have been linked to allergies and headaches. If your child is vegetarian, choose natural protein foods that you know the provenance of, such as beans and lentils, nuts and seeds, eggs and quinoa.

 FASCINATING FACT

Did you know that many cereals, such as granola, contain as much sugar as a chocolate bar?

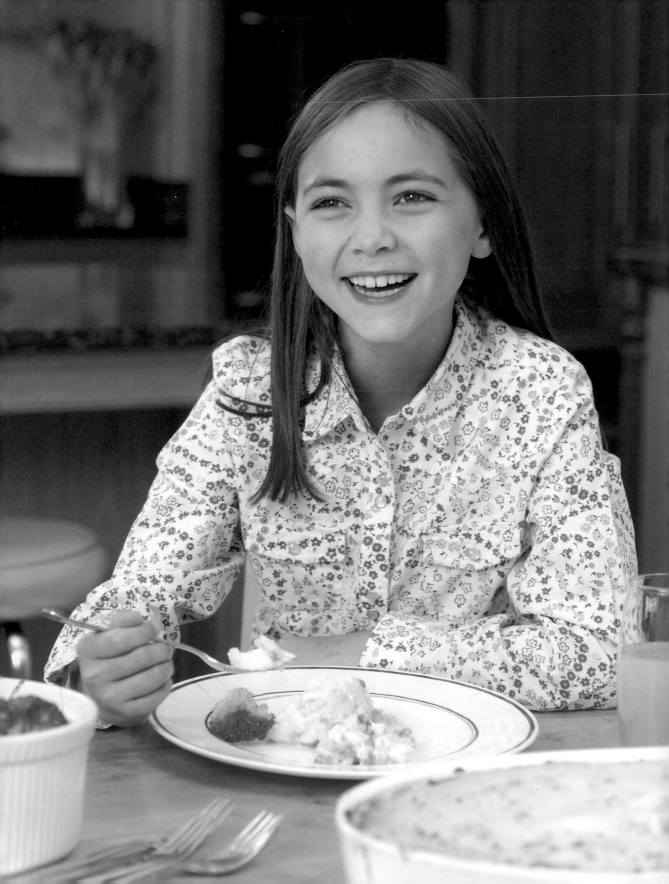

SAVVY SHOPPING

It can be hard to know which foods to choose when shopping, what with media horror stories about hidden nasties and the often misleading advertising claims on supposedly 'healthy' products. Here we have tried to clarify the main issues, from the organic versus non-organic debate, to how to read food labels, so that you can see behind any marketing ploys to determine how healthy a product is, or not. Hopefully, it will help to make the weekly shop less of a minefield.

Organic or not?

Not only does organic food taste better but it is also better for you, with more nutrients and no harmful chemical pesticides, which have been linked to food allergies, behavioural problems and cancers. Plus, it offers better value for money; non-organic produce is pumped up with water so that it appears bigger and, therefore, cheaper, but in fact you are buying less 'product' than the organic version.

In an ideal world we would all buy our food from farmers' markets or reputable local suppliers, secure in the knowledge that our food hadn't been tampered with or sprayed with toxic chemicals. The reality is, however, that for many people organic food is still simply too expensive. If you want to safeguard your family while sticking to a budget, our list of organic priorities should help make shopping easier. The following foods are routinely treated with large amounts of chemicals, so choose organic where possible:

* **Fruit and vegetables that don't need peeling**. These retain more spray residues. When tested, the most toxic fruits and vegetables were found to be: apples, peppers, celery, cherries, grapes, nectarines, peaches, pears, potatoes, berries and spinach.
* **Grains** (such as oats, rice, pasta, flour and products containing them). Grains have a large surface area that is exposed to pesticides.
* **Dairy products, meat and farmed fish**. These contain more saturated fat than organic products, as the animals have less space to exercise, plus the meat contains antibiotic residues from medication routinely given to intensively reared livestock to prevent infection. These upset your body's own gut bacteria balance.

You can still eat organic on a budget if you don't buy the very expensive items (such as imported, out-of-season fruits) but eat cheaper, plant-based foods such as beans and lentils, wholegrains, and seasonal fruit and vegetables. Alternate meat with vegetarian meals for a cheaper, healthier diet. Local, small-scale food produce should also be better quality that intensively produced supermarket stuff, and is much cheaper than organic labelled brands. Plus, buying local reduces air miles.

How to read food labels

Ingredients have to be listed in order of the amount contained in the product, starting with the largest. When a product lists sugar, or one of its many guises (as described below) in the top three ingredients, or if it appears more than once, you know that the product is high in sugar.

Sugar

Sadly, it is increasingly hard to avoid sugar in processed food and snacks these days. It appears in everything from flavoured water to baked beans, often in many different guises to confuse all but the most savvy shoppers. Despite the host of different names and forms for sugars, they all have the same effect: to upset blood sugar balance and adversely affect weight, energy levels and brain function. To work out the sugar content of a product:

Divide the grams of sugar in the product by 4.2 (the number of grams of sugar in a teaspoon). Take, for example, a 35g cereal bar containing 30.3g sugar per 100g, equating to 10.6g per bar – 10.6g divided by 4.2 gives you 2½ teaspoons of sugar per bar.

What is a lot or a little?

Nutrient	A lot (per 100g/3½ oz)	A little (per 100g/3½ oz)
Sugars	10g	2g
Fat	20g	3g
Saturated fat	5g	1g
Fibre	3g	0.5g
Sodium/salt	0.5g/1.25g	0.1g/0.25g

(*to convert sodium to salt multiply by 2.5*)

The following are all types of sugar, and items containing them should be avoided or limited:

brown sugar
corn sweetener
corn syrup
dextrose
fructose
fruit juice concentrates
glucose
high-fructose corn syrup
honey
invert sugar
lactose
malt syrup
maltose
molasses
raw sugar
sucrose
sugar
syrup

Plus artificial sweeteners, which may be low in calories but many have been linked to worrying health concerns.

Low-fat or reduced-fat items

Check the label of low- or reduced-fat items and compare with the original, 'high fat' version, as very often the supposedly healthy alternative can contain much more sugar, salt and/or artificial flavours and fillings in order to compensate for the lack of fat. Common culprits include some low-fat yoghurts, cream cheese, hummus and confectionery.

Choosing fruit juices

If a label says 'pure fruit juice', then it must contain just that: 100 per cent fruit juice. Many juices are made from concentrates, however, and manufacturers are allowed to adjust the water content. This doesn't mean that it has added sugar or other ingredients, just that it won't be as unadulterated as you would expect.

A 'fruit juice drink', on the other hand, is much more adulterated, and may contain as little as 5 per cent fruit juice and the rest water, sugar, artificial sweeteners, flavours and colours. Even pure fruit juice is high in sugar, however, as it is a concentrated source of naturally occurring fruit sugars. You can reduce this by diluting it with water. This also means that you save money, so you can buy better quality, pure fruit juice instead of cheaper, sugary squash or fruit juice drinks.

Flavoured or flavouring?

If you are unsure whether a product is highly processed or natural, see how it is described on the label; labelling laws state that strawberry 'flavoured' yoghurt, for example, must contain real strawberries. Strawberry 'flavouring' or 'flavour', on the other hand, shows that chemical flavouring has been used. Packaging also offers hidden clues: if

the yoghurt contains only artificial 'flavouring', it probably won't have a picture of a strawberry on the pot, as this would be classed as misleading.

Green-light E-number guide

In general, avoid foods that list E numbers in the ingredients list. The following E numbers have been shown to have low or no toxicity, however, and so can be consumed freely.

E number	Name
E414	acacia gum, gum arabic
E355	adipic acid
E503	ammonium carbonates, ammonium hydrogen carbonate, ammonium bicarbonate
E162	beetroot red, betanin(e)
E230	biphenyl (diphenyl or phenyl benzene)
E302	calcium ascorbate
E170	calcium carbonate
E509	calcium chloride
E927B	carbamide (urea)
E330	citric acid
E120	cochineal, carminic acid, carmines
E418	gellan gum
E422	glycerol
E412	guar gum
E507	hydrochloric acid
E410	locust bean gum
E421	mannitol
E461	methyl cellulose
E1200	polydextrose
E357	potassium adipate
E280	propionic acid
E310	propyl gallate
E174	silver
E401	sodium alginate
E451	triphosphates, pentasodium, pentapotassium triphosphate
E967	xylitol

HEALTHY COOKING

You don't need to have any newfangled, expensive gadgets to prepare healthy meals from scratch. These recipes make use of nothing more complicated than a grater, nut mill or coffee grinder and a hand-held blender (although a food processor is useful if you have one, and it will chop and grate foods as well).

It is worth investing in a blender; by blending soups, smoothies and sauces you can conceal all manner of nutritious ingredients from the most paranoid of picky eaters. Food processors that are able to grind nuts and seeds will also allow you to get essential fats into your child easily, or you can grind these in a (cleaned out) coffee-bean grinder or nut mill. As for pans, woks and steamer pans or electric steamer machines all allow you to cook food with the minimum loss of vitamins. We recommend stainless steel pans rather than non-stick ones, as the toxic non-stick coating wears off over time to contaminate your food.

You will notice that these recipes make use of healthy cooking techniques such as steaming, steam-frying (a gentler version of stir-frying using a lid and some liquid to steam food) and poaching, to preserve more nutrients, vitamins and essential fats in the food. Poaching is a brilliant method for cooking fish, as it is gentle enough to protect any delicate essential fats from high temperatures. Simply cover fish in water, stock, milk or a sauce, such as the curried coconut milk in our Coconut Fish Curry on page 104, and simmer gently until the fish is cooked (this depends on the thickness of the fillet, but the flesh should flake easily when pressed).

Frying and deep-frying are avoided, as the high cooking temperature and amount of fat makes these the least healthy cooking methods of all. Grilling or baking food are better options as these avoid direct heat. Meat, fish and vegetables can all be quickly and easily grilled, and it is a healthier option than chargrilling, griddling or barbecuing, all of which cause food to burn and produce toxic acrylamide (a carcinogenic substance found in charred food). You can still enjoy summer barbecues but make sure food is not black on the outside; cook over a more gentle heat, or bake *en papillote* – for this method you simply seal food in a parcel of baking parchment, or baking parchment wrapped in kitchen foil. It is not a good idea to let food come into direct contact with kitchen foil as the aluminium is absorbed by the food, particularly acidic foods such as fruit or tomatoes, or fatty items such as meat or fish.

A microwave oven can be invaluable to save time, but try not to rely on it too heavily, as studies have shown that microwaved vegetables lose fat-soluble vitamins, and the essential omega-3 fats in oily fish are also damaged by the microwave cooking process.

Two-week menu plan

The following menu plan provides a balanced, varied diet for your child, which you can either follow to the letter to make sure you are starting on the right track or you can simply use as a guide or for inspiration.

Most of the menu involves meals made from scratch using the recipes in this book, but although our recipes are designed to be quick and easy, not everyone has time to make fresh meals if both parents are working. If this is the case, don't beat yourself up about it, or give up at the first hurdle. Our Snacks and Lunch Boxes sections (on pages 78 and 83, respectively) include plenty of ready-to-eat bought options such as oatcakes and hummus, and fruit and nuts, plus advice on choosing healthy brands of items such as cereal bars and smoothies. So, if you do not have time for a cookery session with your child, don't worry, you can substitute any of the quicker alternatives from these sections. We have also designed the menu to be as easy as possible, however, so that you can make batches of items for quick meals and snacks later in the week.

Many of our snacks include nuts, but if your child, or their school, avoids nuts, substitute the seeds we suggest instead, which are much less allergenic, or choose another from our Snacks section on page 78.

Puddings

You will notice that we have included an optional pudding every other day. If you have time or if your child is particularly active and has a bigger appetite, then these puddings offer a way to get more fruit, nuts and wholegrains into your child while appealing to their sweet tooth; but these can easily be omitted and saved until weekends or for special occasions.

Drinks

Your child can drink unlimited water (and herbal tea if you can get them to drink it!) but fruit juice should be limited, as even pure fruit juice is a concentrated source of fruit sugars. Aim to give your child no more than one glass a day, and dilute it with some water to offset the sugar load (and cost) even further. If your child currently drinks far more than that, you will have to reduce it gradually, and slowly increase the amount of water in the juice to let your child's taste buds adapt, so that it is eventually half water, half juice. If they are unimpressed by watered-down juice, top up the carton with a splash of water each time you use some, so that as far as they are concerned they are being given undiluted juice straight from the carton. They can also enjoy the fun, colourful and sweet-tasting drinks in our Drinks section on page 142, instead of fizzy drinks and sugary squashes. These can be drunk in moderation – however, if you find that your child is living off these and turning their nose up at meals, then limit them to no more than one per day.

Week one

Day 1
Breakfast Almond Instant Oat Cereal
(page 67)
Snack Vegetable sticks (page 80) with
hummus
Lunch TLT (turkey, lettuce and tomato
sandwich on wholemeal/white 'with added
goodness' bread)
Snack Chocolate Crunchies (page 140), plus
optional piece of fruit if still hungry
Supper Chicken Nuggets (page 98) with
Sweet Potato Wedges (page 116), Big Baked
Beans (page 111) or canned baked beans
and cherry tomatoes
Optional pudding Instant Frozen Yoghurt
(page 126)

Day 2
Breakfast Pick-and-Mix Muesli (page 68)
Snack Apple with handful of walnuts or
sunflower seeds
Lunch Egg mayonnaise and cress sandwich
on wholemeal/white 'with added goodness'
bread or in a toasted wholemeal pitta
bread
Snack Pot or bowl of live natural yogurt with
fresh fruit
Supper Sausage and Pepper Bake (page 89)
with Mini Roasties (page 117)

Day 3
Breakfast Scrambled Eggs (page 77) in a
toasted wholemeal pitta bread (or another,
quicker breakfast if short of time)

Snack Pear and Blueberry Smoothie
(page 73)
Lunch Ham and coleslaw sandwich on
wholemeal/white 'with added goodness'
bread
Snack Chocolate Crunchies (from batch on
day 1), plus optional piece of fruit if still
hungry
Supper Thick Lentil Stew (page 112)
Optional pudding Plum Crumble (page 123)

Day 4
Breakfast Banana Smoothie (page 71)
Snack Two or three plums or apricots plus a
handful of hazelnuts or pumpkin seeds
Lunch Peanut butter or nut/seed butter and
cucumber sandwich on wholemeal/white
'with added goodness' bread
Snack Easiest Ever Flapjacks (page 137), plus
optional piece of fruit if still hungry
Supper Egg Fried Rice (page 107)

Day 5
Breakfast Toast and Nut Butter (page 70)
Snack Fruit smoothie (page 82
Lunch Chicken salad wrap (page 84)
Snack Chocolate Crunchies (from batch
made on day 1), plus optional piece of fruit
if still hungry
Supper Fish Fingers (page 101) with Big
Baked Beans (page 111) or canned baked
beans and steamed broccoli or carrots
Optional pudding Pot or bowl of live
natural yogurt with fresh fruit or Fruit
Compote with Yoghurt (page 125)

Day 6

Breakfast Porridge (page 66) with ground seeds and chopped apple

Snack Celery and Carrot Sailboats (page 80) (older children can have three rough oatcakes with hummus or cottage cheese and cucumber instead)

Lunch (home) Pitta Pizzas (page 108)

Snack Easiest Ever Flapjacks (from batch made on day 4), plus optional piece of fruit if still hungry

Supper Bolognese (page 91) with wholemeal spaghetti

Day 7

Breakfast Boiled Egg(s) (page 76) with toast soldiers

Snack Nectarine (summer) or two clementines (winter) plus a handful of walnuts or pumpkin seeds

Lunch (home) Creamy Cherry Tomato Chicken (page 95) with Sweet Potato Mash (page 117) and steamed sugar snap peas

Snack Fruit smoothie (page 82)

Supper Carrot and Lentil Soup (page 110)

Optional pudding Banana Cheesecake (page 128) with chopped strawberries

Week two

Day 1

Breakfast Jolly Healthy Granola (page 69)

Snack Apple plus a handful of toasted seeds (buy a large tub, from health-food stores, or, far cheaper, make your own following our recipe on page 80, and make a big batch for several snacks during the week)

Lunch Smoked salmon, cream cheese and cucumber sandwich on wholemeal/white 'with added goodness' bread

Snack Banana Cheesecake (leftover from week 1 day 7) with chopped strawberries

Supper Tuna and Fresh Tomato Pasta Sauce (page 102)

Day 2

Breakfast Pear and Blueberry Smoothie (page 73)

Snack Two rough oatcakes with hummus and cucumber sticks

Lunch Tomato Bean Salad (page 86) with Little Gem lettuce leaves and a toasted wholemeal pitta bread

Snack Fistful of ready-to-eat dried apricots or grapes, plus a handful of sunflower seeds or nuts

Supper Chicken and Vegetable Steam-fry (page 97) with brown basmati rice

Optional pudding Banana Cheesecake (if any leftover from week 1 day 7), otherwise a slice of Apple and Almond Tray Bake (page 136), served warm with custard (made with xylitol instead of sugar)

Day 3

Breakfast Toast and Nut Butter (page 70)

Snack Pear plus a handful of toasted seeds (from the batch made on week 2 day 1)

Lunch Titbit Picnic (page 87)

Snack A large slice of Apple and Almond Tray Bake (page 136), plus optional piece of fruit if still hungry

Supper Salmon Teriyaki (page 102) with brown basmati rice or noodles and steam-fried vegetables

Day 4

Breakfast Creamy Raspberry Smoothie (page 72) (summer) or Winter Berry Smoothie (page 75)

Snack Orange or two clementines and a handful of toasted seeds (from the batch made on week 2 day 1)

Lunch Hummus or cottage cheese with four rough oatcakes and vegetable sticks (crudités)

Snack A large slice of Apple and Almond Tray Bake (from the batch made on day 2 or day 3), plus optional piece of fruit if still hungry

Supper Beany Bolognese (page 113) with pasta

Optional pudding Fruit Compote with Yoghurt (page 133)

Day 5

Breakfast Almond Instant Oat Cereal (page 67)

Snack Three apricots or plums (summer) or two clementines (winter) plus a handful of cashew nuts or sunflower seeds

Lunch Chicken salad wrap (page 84)

Snack One slice of Toast and Nut Butter (page 70)

Supper Coconut Fish Curry (page 104) with brown basmati rice

Day 6

Breakfast Poached Egg(s) (page 77) on wholemeal toast

Snack Fruit smoothie (page 82)

Lunch (home) Sweet Potato and Butterbean Soup (page 109) – cook extra for leftovers tomorrow

Snack Blueberries (summer) or clementine segments (winter) with a small pot or bowl of live natural yogurt

Supper Burgers (page 92)

Optional pudding Chocolate Orange Mousse (page 127) with chopped strawberries (summer) or clementine segments (winter)

Day 7

Breakfast Pick-and-Mix Muesli (page 68)

Snack Vegetable sticks (page 80)

Lunch (home) Chicken and Puy Lentil One-Pot Stew (page 94) with Mini Roasties (page 117) or mashed potato

Snack Chocolate Orange Mousse (leftover from day 6) with chopped strawberries (summer) or clementine segments (winter)

Supper Sweet Potato and Butterbean Soup (leftover from day 6)

Breakfasts

Clichéd but true, breakfast really is the most important meal of the day, particularly for children. Their energy stores are at their lowest after a night of fasting when their body has been hard at work growing and carrying out repairs, yet their energy requirements are at their highest, with a whole morning's worth of running around and lessons to face. Yet many of the children we have seen at the Food for the Brain schools were skipping breakfast entirely, or having nothing more than a hastily snatched bowl of sugary cereal. With such unbalanced blood sugar it is no small wonder that so many of them were struggling to concentrate in the classroom. See the Foods to Avoid list for advice on choosing cereals, on page 53.

By providing children with a nutritious breakfast they will have stable energy levels to help them concentrate and behave well at school. Yes, time may be tight in the mornings, with the invariable lost sports kit or battle over teeth brushing, but it is a false economy not to provide your child with a decent breakfast. Here are some breakfast ideas that are low in sugar and rich in wholegrains, fibre and vitamins. They can all be prepared in under five minutes. If your breakfast normally gets forgotten in the struggle to get the children ready, you might like to try them, too.

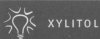 XYLITOL

We use xylitol to sweeten some of the recipes in this chapter. When first using xylitol, increase your daily intake gradually to allow the body to adjust, as large quantities can have a laxative effect. Don't let your child go berserk sweetening their cereal, puddings or drinks with xylitol – they may get a runny tummy as a result. Used in moderation it is a healthy way to include sweet treats in your diet. Do not give to very young children (under two), however, because it is important to get high-calorie, nutrient-dense foods into them as their stomachs are small.

PORRIDGE AND CEREALS

Wholegrain cereals, such as porridge and muesli, are much more filling than the very sugary, refined products marketed at children. Unfortunately, they don't usually come with the added incentive of a free toy or cartoons on the box, but our recipes are tasty enough to help persuade your child to give them a try.

Porridge

Wholegrain oats release their energy slowly – so you avoid the energy rollercoaster that comes from high-GL, sugary, refined cereals. Making porridge from scratch takes no longer than zapping a bowl of instant oat cereal in the microwave, and is far more nutritious, having no sugar, but with extra fibre and vitamins. (For perfect porridge use two parts water to one part oats. Alternatively, use half water, half milk for a creamier consistency.) If using seeds as your topping, limit the flaxseeds (linseeds) to a couple of teaspoons, as these can act as a laxative if consumed with a lot of liquid.

SERVES 1

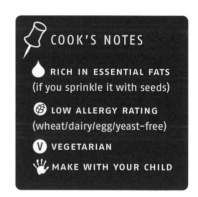

COOK'S NOTES

💧 RICH IN ESSENTIAL FATS
(if you sprinkle it with seeds)

LOW ALLERGY RATING
(wheat/dairy/egg/yeast-free)

Ⓥ VEGETARIAN

✋ MAKE WITH YOUR CHILD

35g (1¼oz) whole porridge oats

225ml (about 7½fl oz) water, or half water, half milk

PLUS, CHOOSE FROM THE FOLLOWING TOPPINGS:

* 1 tsp xylitol and 1 tbsp mixed seeds (flaxseeds, sesame, pumpkin and sunflower seeds). Grind them up and stir in to conceal them from picky eaters, or sprinkle straight from their packets. If you do not grind the flaxseeds, choose pre-cracked ones (from supermarkets and health-food stores), because if they are left whole they can't be digested
* chopped fresh fruit or berries plus 1 tbsp of mixed seeds as above
* drizzle with a spoonful of agave syrup (a low-GL syrup from the cactus, which is hard to come by but delicious; available from health-food stores) and sprinkle with ground cinnamon and/or ginger and chopped apple
* sprinkle of sea salt plus 1 tbsp of mixed seeds as above

Place the oats and water in a pan. Bring to the boil then gently simmer, stirring, until the porridge thickens and the oats soften, about 5 minutes.

Almond Instant Oat Cereal

About as instant as oats get, and as quick to make as a cup of tea. Oats are full of low-GL, slow-release carbohydrates and fibre, and the almonds provide protein and bone-building minerals, calcium and magnesium. Magnesium is known as nature's relaxant, so try this one to calm children down. It is delicious on its own or you can add chopped fresh fruit. If you can't get pre-cracked flaxseeds (linseeds) you can grind whole flaxseeds in order to release their beneficial omega-3 fats and fibre – which also disguises them for fusspots. It's also cheaper.

SERVES 1

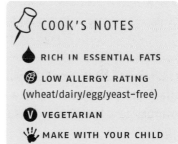

Parent's verdict: 'Loved this – much cheaper than shop-bought brands'

45g (just under 2oz, or 4 tbsp) whole porridge oats

2 tbsp ground almonds

2 heaped tsp xylitol

2 tsp pre-cracked or ground flaxseeds (linseeds)

Place all the ingredients in a bowl and cover with 150ml (5fl oz/¼ pint) boiling water. Stir and leave to thicken for 2 minutes.

COOK'S NOTES

● RICH IN ESSENTIAL FATS

Ⓢ LOW ALLERGY RATING (wheat/dairy/egg/yeast-free)

Ⓥ VEGETARIAN

✋ MAKE WITH YOUR CHILD

FASCINATING FACT

Oats are 'happy food', as they contain a substance called tryptophan, which the brain converts into serotonin – the neurotransmitter that gives us the 'feel-good factor'.

Pick-and-Mix Muesli

Get your child to pick and mix their favourite nuts, seeds and fruit – the ingredients listed here are just a suggestion. If your child won't eat nuts or seeds, grind them first to make them disappear. Serve with live natural yoghurt to get some probiotic bacteria into your child (or soya yoghurt, milk or non-dairy milk) plus fresh fruit. If you like, you could add a few chopped dried apricots or prunes, as these are very rich in antioxidants, and apricots are a good vegan source of iron, but no more than a couple per bowlful to limit the amount of fruit sugar. (Pre-cracked flaxseeds are available from supermarkets and health-food stores.)

75g (3oz) whole porridge oats

2 tsp pumpkin seeds

2 tsp pre-cracked flaxseed (linseeds)

2 tsp flaked almonds

2 tsp desiccated coconut

1 tbsp xylitol

1 tsp ground cinnamon (optional)

½ tsp ground ginger (optional)

live natural yogurt, soya yoghurt, milk or non-dairy milk, to mix

Mix the dried ingredients together and add yoghurt or milk.

SERVES 2

Work out your favourite mixture of nuts and seeds and increase the quantities to make a big batch for easy breakfasts. Store in an airtight container

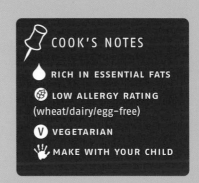

COOK'S NOTES

RICH IN ESSENTIAL FATS

LOW ALLERGY RATING
(wheat/dairy/egg-free)

V VEGETARIAN

MAKE WITH YOUR CHILD

 FASCINATING FACT

A bag of oats is four times cheaper than the same weight of sugar-coated cornflakes, and will fill you up for four times longer.

Jolly Healthy Granola

Did you know that shop-bought cereals like granola-style mueslis and crunchy oat clusters contain some of the highest levels of sugar of all cereals? Many are a third sugar – as much as some chocolate bars! This home-made granola is still sweet, thanks to the xylitol, but it is also sugar-free and low fat, as well as being packed with nuts, seeds and whole grains. Serve with live natural yoghurt and chopped fresh fruit or a few chopped dried apricots and prunes. You can also vary the nuts and seeds:

- 1 tbsp coconut oil, olive oil or butter
- 1 tbsp xylitol
- 50g (2oz) whole oatflakes
- 1 tbsp flaked almonds
- 1 tbsp hazelnuts, roughly chopped
- 1 tbsp pumpkin seeds
- 1 tbsp ground almonds

1. Gently melt the oil or butter in a frying pan with the xylitol, add the oatflakes and stir for 3 minutes, or until they start to go golden and crisp up slightly.
2. Add the flaked almonds and hazelnuts, and stir gently for a further 2 minutes.
3. Remove from the heat and stir in the pumpkin seeds and ground almonds.

SERVES 2
Worth increasing the quantities and making a big batch. Store in an airtight container

> **Parent's verdict:**
> 'A great start to the day. Very filling. Everyone is eating it, although the kids prefer it with dried fruit.'

COOK'S NOTES

- **RICH IN ESSENTIAL FATS**
- **LOW ALLERGY RATING** (wheat/dairy/egg/yeast-free)
- **V VEGETARIAN**
- **MAKE WITH YOUR CHILD**

FASCINATING FACT

Your brain is 60 per cent fat, so make sure that it is made up of the right fats; the essential fatty acid omega-3 is critical for brain development and function in children. Make sure they eat flaxseeds (linseeds), pumpkin and hemp seeds, and walnuts, as well as oily fish or eggs from chickens fed on flaxseeds (and consider a fish oil supplement).

Toast and Nut Butter

Parent's verdict: 'I still can't get my child to eat wholemeal bread but they will eat hazelnut butter on "all-in-one" white bread "with added goodness". A real change from the white toast with golden syrup that they used to eat!'

SERVES 1

Toast is one of the most popular and easiest breakfasts, but make sure you use wholegrain bread to give your child fibre and slow-releasing carbohydrate. We found that the Food for the Brain children who baulked at 'bread with bits in' were successfully duped by the new range of 'all-in-one' white breads, which have had the goodness added back in. Or serve rye bread or 3–4 rough oatcakes, which don't even need toasting. Top with a spread that contains protein to slow down the release of sugar from the carbohydrate in the bread. Nut butter is perfect, as the nuts provide minerals and essential fats as well as protein. Top with banana slices for an extra-filling version. When choosing nut butters go for unsweetened, unsalted brands; look in health-food stores if you cannot find them in supermarkets.

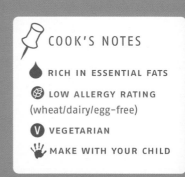

COOK'S NOTES

🔸 RICH IN ESSENTIAL FATS

🌐 LOW ALLERGY RATING
(wheat/dairy/egg-free)

Ⓥ VEGETARIAN

🖐 MAKE WITH YOUR CHILD

> 1–2 slices wholegrain bread or pumpernickel-style rye bread
>
> peanut butter, or another nut butter such as cashew, hazelnut or almond, or pumpkin seed butter

Toast the bread and spread with nut butter.

BREAKFAST SMOOTHIES

These smoothies are all designed to replace a sit-down meal if your child has neither the time nor appetite for breakfast in the morning. They also make excellent snacks and can go in a chilled lunch box. You will notice that they all contain seeds, as this is a brilliant way to get these essential fat-, protein- and mineral-rich foods into your child's diet on the sly, to boost brain function.

Banana Smoothie

This thick, naturally sweet smoothie tastes like a milkshake and takes moments to prepare. Seeds contain essential fats, which help eye and brain development. You can also add a handful of strawberries or blueberries. Grind the sunflower seeds using a blender or coffee grinder or blend them with the rest of the smoothie to save time, although if you do this some little nibs will remain.

1 tbsp sunflower seeds, ground

1 banana

3 tbsp live natural yoghurt

about 90ml (3fl oz) milk or juice, if necessary

Using a hand-held blender or a liquidiser, blend all the ingredients together until smooth, adding just enough milk or juice to loosen the mixture to a drinking consistency.

SERVES 1 (SHORT GLASS)

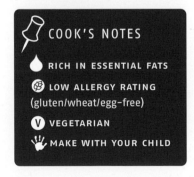

Parent's verdict: 'A great way to get the kids eating fruit.' Children's verdict: 'Absolutely lovely.'

COOK'S NOTES

RICH IN ESSENTIAL FATS

LOW ALLERGY RATING (gluten/wheat/egg-free)

V VEGETARIAN

MAKE WITH YOUR CHILD

Creamy Raspberry Smoothie

Parent's verdict: 'Really healthy and the children don't even know it! All three of mine enjoyed these smoothies and they won't have shop-bought ones again!'

Tested by Shelley, aged 10. Verdict: 'Can't get enough of these!'

A dairy-free smoothie that is very rich and creamy thanks to the tahini (sesame seed paste). It is packed with antioxidant flavonoids and vitamin C from the raspberries, to provide brain energy and help fight infections, and protein and minerals from the tahini – a good meal in a glass for reluctant breakfast eaters. Vary the flavour by using strawberries or blueberries instead of raspberries, or a mixture. Add a banana to make it more filling and even thicker – in which case you won't need to sweeten it with as much xylitol.

SERVES 1 (SHORT GLASS)

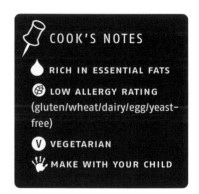

COOK'S NOTES

◌ RICH IN ESSENTIAL FATS

◉ LOW ALLERGY RATING (gluten/wheat/dairy/egg/yeast-free)

Ⓥ VEGETARIAN

✋ MAKE WITH YOUR CHILD

   75g (3oz) raspberries
   1 tbsp tahini
   3 tsp xylitol (or to taste)
   100ml (3½fl oz) water

Using a hand-held blender or a liquidiser, blend all the ingredients together.

Pear and Blueberry Smoothie

A real brain-boosting meal in a glass, thanks to the vitamin
C in the blueberries and the zinc in the seeds, both of which
help the brain turn glucose into energy, for school fuel.
Grind the seeds using a blender or coffee grinder or blend
them with the smoothie to save time, although if you do this
some little nibs will remain.

SERVES 1

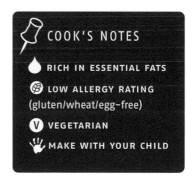

Parent's verdict:
'We're completely
converted to
smoothies now.'

1 tbsp sunflower or pumpkin seeds, ground

1 small pear, cored and roughly chopped

75g (3oz) (about 3 heaped tbsp) blueberries

3 tbsp live natural yoghurt

about 90ml (3fl oz) milk, juice or water

Using a hand-held blender or a liquidiser, blend all the
ingredients together, adding just enough milk, juice or water
to loosen the mixture to a drinking consistency.

COOK'S NOTES

💧 **RICH IN ESSENTIAL FATS**

⊗ **LOW ALLERGY RATING**
(gluten/wheat/egg-free)

Ⓥ **VEGETARIAN**

🖐 **MAKE WITH YOUR CHILD**

 FASCINATING FACT

Probiotic drinks and yoghurts may be branded as 'active
health' drinks but many contain up to 80 per cent more
sugar, weight for weight, than cola! Choose live, natural
yoghurt, miso or tempeh for unsweetened sources of
probiotic, or friendly, bacteria.

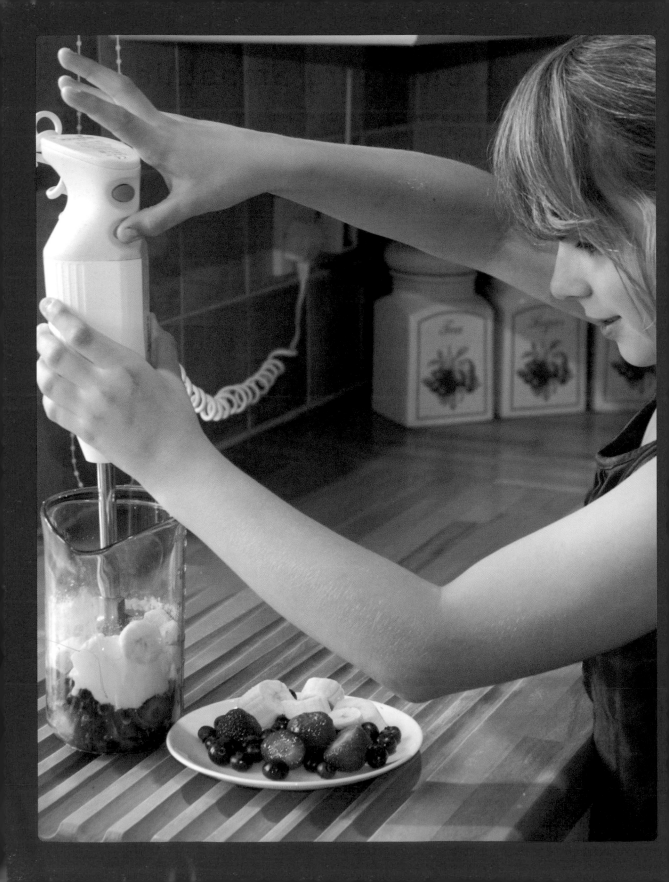

Winter Berry Smoothie

When summer fruits are out of season use bags of frozen berries from supermarkets for a winter vitamin-C fix to help your child's brain turn glucose into energy, and give their immune system a boost, helping to stop them picking up classroom coughs and colds. Grind the seeds in a blender or coffee grinder or blend them with the rest of the smoothie to save time, although this way some little nibs may remain. Leave the berries to defrost for a few minutes or overnight if your blender struggles with fully frozen ones.

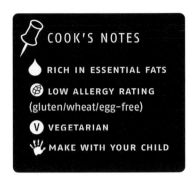

COOK'S NOTES

💧 RICH IN ESSENTIAL FATS

⊗ LOW ALLERGY RATING
(gluten/wheat/egg-free)

Ⓥ VEGETARIAN

✋ MAKE WITH YOUR CHILD

- 1 tbsp seeds (such as a mixture of linseeds, pumpkin, sesame and sunflower seeds), ground
- 100g (3½oz) frozen mixed berries, or fresh ones in the summer
- 1 banana
- 100g (3½oz) live natural yoghurt
- 1 tbsp xylitol, or to taste

Using a hand-held blender or a liquidiser, blend the ingredients together until smooth. This is very thick smoothie, so it can either be eaten with a spoon, or loosened with a little water to make it easier to drink.

FASCINATING FACT

Being just 3 per cent dehydrated can impact your mental and physical performance by as much as 10 per cent! So drink the equivalent of eight glasses of water a day. Fresh fruit and vegetables all contribute to your water intake.

EGGS

Choose eggs for a brilliantly brainy breakfast. They are not only an excellent source of protein to help your child grow, but they are also rich in B vitamins, which help balance mood and energy, and zinc, which has been shown to be hugely important in helping boost memory and brain function. The yolks also contain special fats called phospholipids, which are used to connect brain cells to keep your child's brain performing at top speed.

Buy organic or, at the very least, free range eggs; not only preferable from the point of view of the chicken's welfare, but also because the eggs are richer in nutrients than those from poor old battery-farmed hens. Many supermarkets now sell omega-3-rich eggs from chickens fed on flaxseeds (linseeds), which is a good way to get omega-3 oils into your child if they do not like fish or are vegetarian.

Eggs are best cooked lightly, so as not to damage the phospholipids in the yolk. This means soft boiling, poaching and lightly scrambling them.

Old advice used to be to limit eggs to no more than three per week because of their high cholesterol content. In fact, the body is able to adjust for a high intake of cholesterol through the diet by down-regulating its own cholesterol production, thereby keeping levels in check.

Boiled Eggs

Serve with toast 'soldiers' made from wholemeal bread, 'all-in-one' white bread 'with added goodness' or rye bread. Don't bother buttering the toast as the yolk contains enough fat and flavour that you don't need extra.

SERVES 1

1 or 2 free range or organic eggs, pricked with an egg pricker (optional)

1 Bring a pan of water to a slow boil and gently place the eggs into the pan. Leave to boil gently for 8 minutes.
2 Remove from the pan and quickly run under cold water to prevent them cooking further.

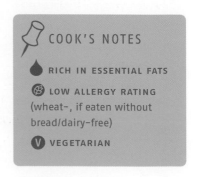

COOK'S NOTES

RICH IN ESSENTIAL FATS

LOW ALLERGY RATING (wheat-, if eaten without bread/dairy-free)

V VEGETARIAN

Scrambled Eggs

Comfort food for cold mornings. Serve with wholemeal or 'all-in-one' white 'with added goodness' toast, rye bread or even in a toasted wholemeal pitta bread.

SERVES 1

2 free range or organic eggs

freshly ground black pepper

pinch of sea salt

2 tsp coconut oil, olive oil or butter

1 Beat the eggs with the pepper and salt.
2 Heat the oil in a small pan over a gentle heat and pour in the beaten eggs.
3 Slowly stir the eggs with a wooden spoon, scraping along the base of the pan as they cook. Remove from the heat as soon as the eggs are almost set but still slightly moist.

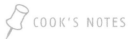

COOK'S NOTES

RICH IN ESSENTIAL FATS

LOW ALLERGY RATING (wheat-free, if eaten without bread/dairy-free if not using butter)

V VEGETARIAN

Poached Eggs

Much healthier than fried eggs, which are very fatty and cooked at such a high temperature that the brain-boosting phospholipids in the egg yolk get damaged. Serve on wholemeal or 'all-in-one' white 'with added goodness' toast or wheat-free rye bread or oatcakes.

SERVES 1

1 or 2 medium or large free range or organic eggs

1 Half-fill a frying pan with boiling water and bring to a gentle simmer (you should just be able to see small bubbles forming on the base of the pan).
2 Crack the eggs into the pan, taking care not to puncture the yolks. They should be just covered with water – if not, carefully add a little more boiling water.
3 Let the eggs cook in the simmering water for 4 minutes, spooning water gently over the yolks to help them to cook then carefully lift out the eggs using a slotted spoon.

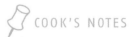

COOK'S NOTES

RICH IN ESSENTIAL FATS

LOW ALLERGY RATING (wheat-free, if eaten without bread/dairy-free)

V VEGETARIAN

Snacks

A mid-morning and mid-afternoon snack will help your child's blood sugar stay balanced to keep their energy levels even. Choosing low-sugar, low-GL snacks that combine protein and some slow-release carbohydrate (like fruit or whole grains) will help avoid the hyperactive highs and lethargic lows that you may have witnessed after giving your child sugary drinks, biscuits or sweets.

Snacks also present another opportunity to get some extra fruit, vegetables, nuts and seeds into your child. Here are some nutritious, easy-to-eat options that you can also include in lunch boxes. There are also plenty of healthy sweet snack ideas in the Cakes, Biscuits and Sweets section on page 133.

Fruit

Choose fresh fruit over dried, and opt for low-sugar ones such as apples, pears, berries, plums, apricots, oranges and peaches, rather than bananas, grapes and tropical fruit, which are naturally much sweeter. Best eaten with a handful of nuts or seeds or some yoghurt, to provide protein to slow down the release of sugars in the fruit.

Dried apricots

Although dried fruit is a concentrated source of fruit sugars, bags of dried fruit make very handy snacks that go down well with most children. Apricots are particularly good as they are very rich in the antioxidant vitamin beta-carotene and also iron. Go for ready-pitted ones that are unsulphured, as the preservative sulphur dioxide is linked to allergies and asthma.

Nuts

If your child's school allows nuts, these make a convenient and incredibly nutritious snack, as they are jam-packed with protein, essential fats and minerals to fuel them through lessons. Choose raw, unsalted nuts if your child will eat them, and go for different types such as almonds, walnuts, brazil nuts, hazelnuts, cashew nuts and pecan nuts, not just the perennial peanut.

Seeds

You can carry bags of seeds in your handbag, or put a sachet into lunch boxes. Seeds are a good source of protein for energy, plus essential fats and zinc to feed the brain. Sunflower and pumpkin seeds are the most popular and a good size for nibbling. Like nuts, go for raw if your child will eat them, to make the most of the essential fats, but if they find these bland, you can buy packets of toasted, seasoned seeds, or make your own, using the recipe on page 80.

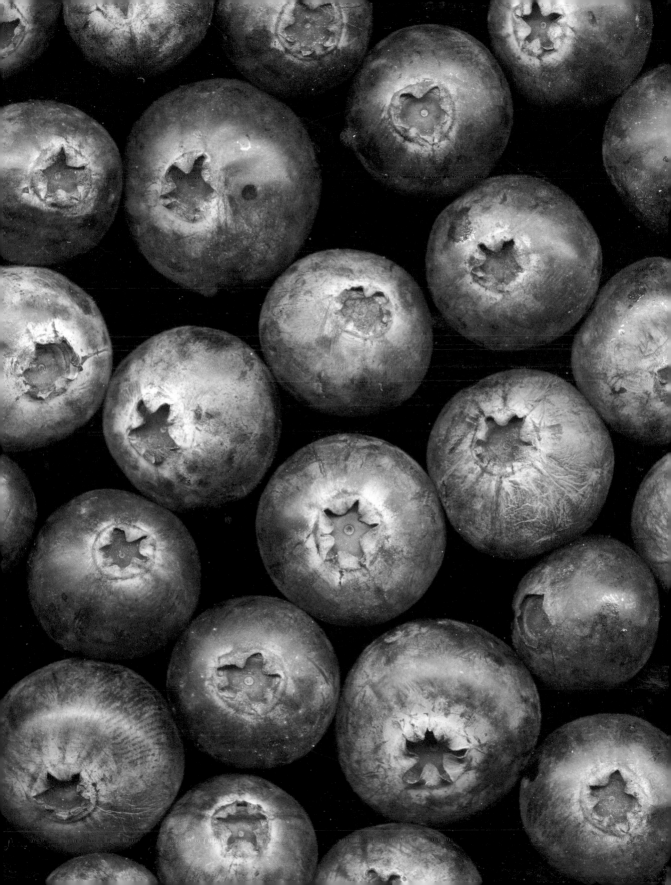

Toasted Seeds

These crunchy, salty seeds are a good alternative to crisps and provide essential omegas-3 and 6 instead of the harmful saturated and trans-fats found in fried potatoes. They are also far more filling, as they contain protein instead of starchy, high-GL carbohydrate.

SERVES 12

Make in bulk for convenient snacks, and store in an airtight container. Make a fresh batch each week

200g (7oz) seeds (try mixing sunflower and pumpkin seeds)

a drizzle (about 2 tsp) of tamari (wheat-free soy sauce) or soy sauce, or a sprinkle of sea salt, to taste

1 Gently toast the seeds in a dry frying pan for 2–3 minutes, or until they start to turn crisp and golden. Stir in the tamari, soy or salt just before you remove the pan from the heat.
2 Leave to cool before eating.

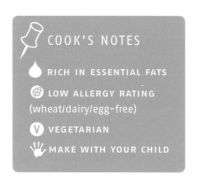

COOK'S NOTES

RICH IN ESSENTIAL FATS

LOW ALLERGY RATING (wheat/dairy/egg-free)

V VEGETARIAN

MAKE WITH YOUR CHILD

Vegetable sticks

Chopped raw vegetables, or crudités, are easy to eat and fun to dip into pots of hummus, guacamole, cottage cheese, cream cheese or tomato salsa. Most children like the texture and crunch of raw vegetables, so if they spurn cooked veg, don't worry, as eating them raw provides even more vitamins anyway. Don't just opt for carrot and cucumber sticks; try to go for a rainbow of colours to ensure your child gets a whole range of phyto (plant) nutrients. Try peppers (not green, which are too bitter raw), celery, cherry tomatoes, baby corn, sugar snap peas, radishes, baby spring onions, and even broccoli florets.

Celery and Carrot Sailboats

Fiona's husband Nick has very fond memories of making these edible sailboats when he was little. They are a novel way to get some raw vegetables into younger children, and the filling provides protein.

Cut a stick of celery into pieces each about 5cm (2in) long. Spread a spoonful of peanut butter, hummus, cream cheese or cottage cheese into the hollow of each one. Cut a slice of carrot into a long triangle to look like a sail and stick upright into the filling.

Oatcakes

Because they contain less gluten than wheat, oatcakes are easier to digest than bread. They also contain more fibre to help digestion, and fill you up for longer. Choose the rough-milled ones as these have a lower GL as the more coarsely ground grains take longer to be broken down. Spread two or three with cottage cheese, cream cheese, hummus or nut butter (all of which contain protein to balance blood sugar) for an easy snack. Nut butter or sugar-free jam topped with banana slices is also delicious on oatcakes.

Rice cakes

Rice is a high-GL carbohydrate as it contains a lot of starch that readily converts to sugar. This means that rice cakes will not balance blood sugar as successfully as oatcakes, which take longer to digest, nor are they as filling. They are a good gluten-free option for children with allergies, however, and are easy to eat when children are out. Spread the rice cake with some protein to slow down the sugar release from the rice – such as hummus, cottage cheese, cream cheese or nut butter. Brown rice is also a good source of B vitamins, needed to keep your child alert and in a good mood.

Toast

A slice of toasted rye bread or wholemeal bread (or even 'all-in-one' white bread 'with added goodness') makes a no-fuss snack. Spread with some protein-rich nut butter or hummus and slice into fingers. Rye bread is particularly nutritious as it is made of wholegrains and is easier to digest, and fills you up for longer than wheat bread. Cut it very thinly, as it is so much denser than standard, wheat loaves, or buy pre-sliced pumpernickel-style rye bread.

Yoghurt with fruit

The combination of fruit (slow-release, low-GL carbohydrate) and yoghurt (protein) makes this a blood-sugar balancing, energy-boosting snack. Choose live natural yogurt, as it will have no added sugar and contains the beneficial probiotic bacteria that help digestion and fight bugs. Choose low-sugar fruits such as apples, pears, berries, apricots, plums, oranges and peaches rather than high-sugar bananas, grapes and tropical fruit. You can pop a tub of berries or chopped fruit in your child's lunch box for them to mix or dip into their yoghurt.

Fruit smoothies

Make your own fresh smoothies using fruit and live natural yoghurt for a perfectly balanced snack containing slow-release, low-GL carbohydrate from the fruit, and low-fat protein from the yoghurt. See the recipes in the Breakfast Smoothies section on page 71, or experiment with your own combinations. If your child cannot eat dairy products you can substitute banana, thinned with a little water or apple juice, tahini, again thinned with water, or coconut milk to get the same creamy consistency. You can also buy smoothies that contain no added sugar and plenty of fresh fruit these days, which make useful snacks for lunch boxes or when you are out.

Sugar-free cereal bars

There are lots of cereal and muesli bars on the market these days, but most of them contain alarming amounts of sugar (as much as a third), so that they rival chocolate bars for sweetness. Look in health-food stores or the healthy-eating section of supermarkets for some of the healthier options that are becoming increasingly available. Choose one that has little or no added sugar, syrup, honey, fructose or sweetened dried fruit, as all of these upset blood sugar balance. Look for ones made of wholegrains like oats,

which are sweetened with a little dried fruit, plus nuts and/or seeds for protein to slow down the release of sugar. Fruitus bars by Lyme Regis Foods are one of the best brands available in the UK.

Flapjacks

Like cereal and muesli bars, flapjacks are usually just as high in sugar as biscuits and chocolate bars. You can make your own, healthier version very easily, however, using the recipe for the Easiest Ever Flapjacks on page 137 of the Cakes, Biscuits and Sweets section.

Chocolate

A little chocolate once in a while is not going to hurt anyone, but avoid cheap milk and white chocolate, as it has extra sugar to make up for the lack of cocoa solids. Good-quality chocolate that has a relatively high cocoa solid content (from 50–60 per cent upwards) tastes infinitely superior and is lower in sugar. Plus, it also contains iron and magnesium – a natural relaxant mineral. Chocolate-covered nuts or seeds are another good compromise – the protein in the nuts helps to slow down the speedy sugar release from the chocolate.

Lunch Boxes

If you want to your child to enjoy balanced energy levels and be able to settle down at school, you need to give them the right foods and drinks. Lunch boxes are tricky to get right, however. Make them too obviously healthy and your child will turn their nose up at them (or, as Fiona's little sister Olivia used to do, hide the sandwiches in their PE bag, only to be discovered later with a term's worth of mould on). But pander too much to their tastes and your child will yo-yo between hyperactivity and lethargy on a blood-sugar rollercoaster ride. The harmful additives and preservatives found in most processed foods aimed at children have also been linked to behavioural problems, asthma and allergies.

Lots of the children's lunch boxes at the Food for the Brain schools were found to contain the following recipe for a poor attention span and hyperactivity:

* **White bread sandwich**
* **Chocolate bar or biscuit**
* **Packet of crisps**
* **Fizzy drink or sugary squash**

This nutrient-poor, additive-, fat- and sugar-laden collection of foods may go down well in the playground but it is no wonder that so many of these children suffered from behavioural problems and/or learning difficulties. In order to avoid 'hiding healthy food in the PE bag' scenarios, the solution is to make gradual changes, swapping crisps for fruit one week, and chocolate for a cereal bar or healthy home-made flapjack the next, adding in another change each week to get your child used to the new foods without making any drastic dietary overhauls.

The Menu Plan on page 61 includes a full two weeks' worth of lunch box ideas, but if you are creating your own, you can use the following guidelines as a healthy template:

* **A piece of fruit or chopped raw vegetables** – plus a handful of nuts or seeds, a yoghurt or a dip such as hummus, cottage cheese or cream cheese to provide protein for a more sustaining, low-GL snack, if possible.
* **Another snack item** See the Snacks list on page 78, and the Cakes, Biscuits and Sweets section on page 133 for some ideas for healthy treats.
* **Water**, or diluted, sugar-free, pure fruit juice. (See our advice for Choosing Fruit Juices on page 59.)
* **Main lunch item, such as a sandwich, wrap or salad** Ideally sandwiches should be made with wholegrain bread (such as wholemeal bread or pitta bread), rye bread or with oatcakes. Don't buy bread simply labelled 'brown' – it is likely to be white bread that has simply been dyed brown! Make sure the label says 'wholemeal'. Or choose an 'all-in-one' white bread 'with added goodness'. Include some protein in sandwiches and salads (such as chicken, turkey, eggs, tuna, salmon or hummus) and vegetables (salad or raw vegetables chopped into bite-sized portions). For

fillings like cream cheese, cottage cheese, coleslaw, tuna or egg mayo and nut butter, there is no need to add extra butter, but for 'drier' fillings, you can use a little butter or margarine (choose one that says that it contains no hydrogenated fats, partially hydrogenated fats or trans-fats).

Here are some healthy sandwich fillings and salad ideas to get you started:

* Smoked salmon, cream cheese and cucumber on wholemeal/'all-in-one' white bread or rye bread.
* Oatcakes and vegetable sticks (crudités) with hummus or cottage cheese dip.
* Wholemeal pitta bread stuffed with soy and sesame seasoned tuna, with lettuce and cherry tomatoes.
* Egg mayonnaise on wholemeal/'all-in-one' white bread with cress, alfalfa sprouts (which look and taste very similar to cress) or cucumber slices.
* Peanut butter (or other nut/seed butter) and cucumber on wholemeal/'all-in-one' white bread.
* Cottage cheese and prawns on wholemeal/'all-in-one' white bread or in wholemeal pitta bread.
* Chicken salad wrap. Sliced chicken, with a mixed salad, wrapped in a tortilla.
* TLT (turkey, lettuce and tomato on wholemeal/'all-in-one' white bread or in wholemeal pitta bread).
* Ham (unprocessed and not made from reconstituted meat, but off the bone from the deli) and coleslaw on wholemeal/

'all-in-one' white bread or in wholemeal pitta bread.
* Tomato Bean Salad (see page 86).
* Titbit Picnic (for picky eaters) (see page 87).

 FASCINATING FACT

'Brown bread' is just white bread dyed brown; unless it says 'wholemeal' on the label, it won't be made from wholegrain flour.

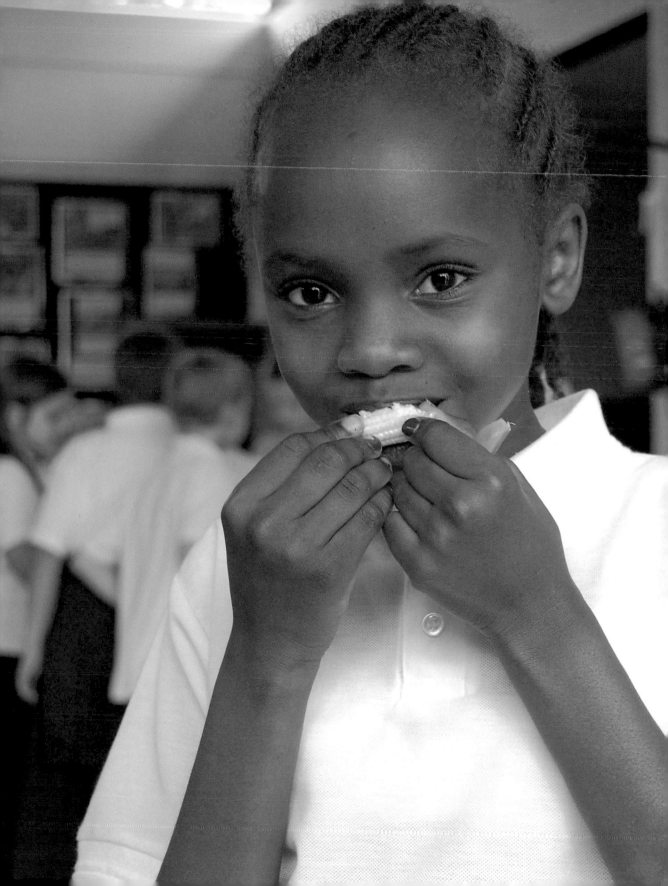

Tomato Bean Salad

This can be thrown together in a couple of minutes flat – or stirred together by your child. It is packed with eyesight-helping carotenoids from the brightly coloured vegetables. The olives provide a strong, salty flavour for older children or those with more adventurous taste buds, but could easily be omitted. You could also add diced red onion and celery. Serve with Little Gem lettuce leaves so that the salad can be spooned into the leaves and eaten with fingers, as well as with a toasted wholemeal pitta bread.

1 × 410g (14½oz) can mixed pulses, drained and rinsed

1 red, yellow or orange pepper, diced

about 6 cherry tomatoes, diced

about 8 pitted black olives, roughly chopped (optional)

2 tbsp good-quality tomato-based pasta sauce, or sun-dried tomato paste, or 1 tbsp pesto (enough to coat)

freshly ground black pepper, to taste

handful of fresh basil leaves, torn (optional)

Mix all the ingredients together, taste and adjust the seasoning if necessary.

Parent's verdict: 'Nice mixture and tasty. A great lunch-box filler.'

Tested by the Burgess children: 'We didn't used to like tomatoes but this is yummy.'

 COOK'S NOTES

 LOW ALLERGY RATING (gluten/wheat/dairy/egg-free)

V VEGETARIAN

MAKE WITH YOUR CHILD

Titbit Picnic (for picky eaters)

Providing a selection of tempting finger foods to nibble at, instead of one main item, works well with children who tend to dissect their food or quickly lose interest. If your child likes each food to be kept separate, put items in individual plastic containers. You can adapt our suggestions to your child's tastes while trying to get in as many vegetables as possible and some protein – try cucumber and carrot sticks instead of the pepper and baby corn, for example. You can spice up the chicken for more adventurous palates by sprinkling it with mild curry powder or dried fajita spices prior to cooking.

SERVES 1

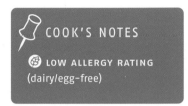

COOK'S NOTES

LOW ALLERGY RATING
(dairy/egg-free)

1 skinless, boneless chicken breast

handful of cherry tomatoes

½ yellow or orange pepper, sliced into strips

handful of baby corn

mini wholemeal pitta bread, toasted or 3 rough oatcakes

mini pot of hummus

salt and freshly ground black pepper

1 To make chicken goujons, slice the chicken breast into strips and stir-fry for 5–6 minutes in a little oil until cooked (cut a piece in half and check that there is no pink flesh and that the juices run clear). Sprinkle with salt and pepper.
2 Serve with the other ingredients, either arranged separately on one plate or in individual bowls.

Family Meals

The recipes in this section have been designed to be suitable for the whole family, to encourage you to sit down and eat together. Sharing a meal with your child is the best way to keep an eye on their eating habits (and table manners), and to set a good example by putting your money where your mouth is and eating all your broccoli or fish, or whatever food it is that they are spurning. Plus, cooking one dish for everyone is far quicker than preparing separate meals, and it saves on washing up.

We have also tried to provide a range of dishes to suit every taste, so if you are just starting to wean your child off nuggets, smiley potato faces and spaghetti hoops, our home-made Chicken Nuggets or Fish Fingers, for example, should help smooth the transition to healthier foods. Likewise, if you have slightly older children, or are fortunate enough to have easy eaters, the Chicken and Puy Lentil One-Pot Supper is absolutely delicious, and is suitable for serving at a supper party for your own friends. Many of the recipes contain serving suggestions to try to get extra vegetables into your child, but don't despair if they refuse to eat them – there are vegetables integral to most of the dishes anyway.

MEAT AND POULTRY

There are family favourites here such as Bolognese, plus some child-friendly dishes such as Burgers and Chicken Nuggets. All of them have been given a nutrition makeover to make them packed with vitamins, minerals and fibre, without compromising on the taste that makes them so popular.

If you compare the Bolognese, for example, to one in a standard recipe book, you will see that ours uses far more vegetables, to increase the nutrient content. Likewise, our Chicken Nuggets are a far cry from the reconstituted meat and the highly processed, artificially coloured coating seen in ones from fast-food outlets or as frozen ready meals. The quality of the meat you buy will also affect the nutrient content of these recipes. Meat that has been reared organically, or not intensively farmed, will be lower in fat and richer in nutrients – the cheapest and most reputable sources are direct from the producer at farmers' markets, or try a good-quality butchers (see the Organic or Not? section on page 57).

Sausage and Pepper Bake

Look for good-quality sausages with a high meat content and avoid ones that are full of additives and fillers. Labels that read simply 'sausages' are only required to contain 32 per cent meat, whereas those labelled 'pork sausages' must contain at least 42 per cent. The best place to find good bangers is at farmers' markets, direct from the producers or from good-quality butchers. Serve with Mini Roasties (see page 117) or baked sweet potatoes. You can prepare this dish in advance and pop it into the oven an hour before you want to eat, or reheat leftovers.

6 peppers (mixed colours), deseeded and sliced into long, thin strips

3 red onions, sliced into long strips (or replace with another pepper)

2 × 400g (14oz) cans chopped tomatoes

5 tbsp tomato purée

12 sausages (choose gluten-free ones without breadcrumbs or cereal fillers, if necessary)

sea salt and freshly ground black pepper

1 Preheat the oven to 190°C/375°F/Gas 5.
2 Place the chopped peppers and onions in a large, shallow casserole dish, stir in the tomatoes and purée, and season with a little salt. Place the sausages on top.
3 Cook for about 1 hour, or until the sausages are cooked and the vegetables are soft. Turn the sausages halfway through cooking.
4 Season generously with black pepper.

SERVES 6

Parent's verdict: 'We all loved this.'

Tested by: Shelley, aged 12. Verdict: 'Scrummy, we want it every day.'

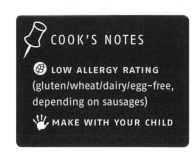

COOK'S NOTES

LOW ALLERGY RATING (gluten/wheat/dairy/egg-free, depending on sausages)

MAKE WITH YOUR CHILD

Sausages with Golden Mash and Baked Beans

Sweet potatoes mash down to a naturally creamy consistency without the need to add extra butter or milk. They are also more nutritious than white potatoes as the orange flesh contains lots of antioxidant vitamins like beta-carotene and vitamin E, although normal spuds can be used instead. When choosing beans, some of the organic brands of baked beans are sweetened with a little apple juice instead of sugar and have fewer additives. Failing that, go for bog-standard beans, not the ones with no added sugar, as these contain artificial sweeteners and fillers that can be even more harmful than sugar. Prick the sausages with a fork before cooking so that the excess fat will drip out while they cook.

SERVES 4

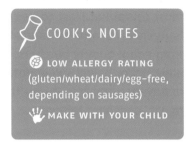

COOK'S NOTES

LOW ALLERGY RATING
(gluten/wheat/dairy/egg-free, depending on sausages)

MAKE WITH YOUR CHILD

8 good-quality sausages with a high meat content, pricked (choose gluten-free ones without breadcrumbs or cereal fillers, if necessary)

2 medium–large sweet potatoes, peeled and finely sliced

2 carrots, peeled and finely sliced

1 tsp Marigold Reduced Salt Vegetable Bouillon powder, or sea salt to taste

2 × 410g (14½oz) cans baked beans or 1 quantity of Big Baked Beans, to serve 4 (see page 111)

freshly ground black pepper

1 Grill or oven-cook the sausages according to the packet instructions.
2 Meanwhile, steam the sweet potato and carrot for about 12–15 minutes, or until soft, before mashing together. Season lightly with the bouillon powder or the sea salt and keep warm while you heat up the beans.

Bolognese

We have used far more vegetables than usual to make this Bolognese sauce a very good source of fibre, vitamins and minerals. Blend them so that they are disguised in the thick sauce if necessary. Serve with wholemeal or wheat/gluten-free spaghetti or a baked potato or sweet potato, and peas. Or you can top the Bolognese with Sweet Potato Mash (see page 117) to turn it into an instant shepherd's pie of sorts. Good-quality, lean beef is an excellent source of protein, to allow the brain to make neurotransmitters to send messages.

SERVES 4

Parent's verdict: 'A healthy meal, easy and quick to make.'

Tested by: Hope, aged 10. Verdict: 'Love it!'

2 tsp coconut oil or olive oil

1 onion, diced

2 garlic cloves, crushed

200g (7oz) mushrooms, brushed clean or wiped with kitchen paper and sliced

1 carrot, grated or 1 pepper, diced

450g (1lb) lean, good-quality beef or lamb mince

1 × 400g (14oz) can chopped tomatoes

3 tbsp tomato purée

3 tsp Marigold Reduced Salt Vegetable Bouillon powder, or sea salt to taste

1 tsp dried oregano, or to taste

freshly ground black pepper

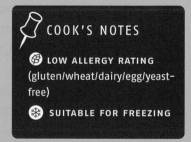

COOK'S NOTES

LOW ALLERGY RATING (gluten/wheat/dairy/egg/yeast-free)

SUITABLE FOR FREEZING

1 Heat the oil in a large saucepan or stockpot and sweat the onion, garlic, mushrooms and carrot or pepper for about 5 minutes to soften. Remove from the pan and set to one side.
2 Add the mince to the pan and fry for 2 minutes to brown the meat (if the mince is fatty scoop off any excess with a teaspoon), then stir in the vegetable mixture and remaining ingredients. Cover and simmer for 5–10 minutes, or until the vegetables are soft and the sauce has thickened. Season with black pepper.

Burgers

This recipe uses lamb, which is the least likely meat to cause allergies and is a good source of brain-fuelling protein and minerals. You could also use beef or turkey mince. The onion used in this recipe is invisible once cooked, so fusspots won't notice it, but it provides anti-inflammatory power to help asthma, eczema and other inflammatory conditions. Delicious with lettuce, tomato and a dollop of ketchup in wholemeal pitta bread rather than refined, white buns, or you can serve with salad, baked beans and Sweet Potato Wedges (see page 116).

SERVES 3–4
(MAKES 6–8 BURGERS)

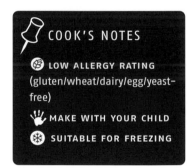

Parent's verdict:
'Lovely and healthy.
Great to know what
is in the burgers.
Very tasty.'

500g (1lb 2oz) lamb mince

1 very small red onion, finely diced

½ tsp ground cumin

½ tsp ground coriander

1 tsp sea salt

lots of freshly ground black pepper

2 tbsp finely chopped fresh flat-leaf parsley

a little coconut oil or olive oil, for frying

COOK'S NOTES

⊗ LOW ALLERGY RATING
(gluten/wheat/dairy/egg/yeast-free)

✋ MAKE WITH YOUR CHILD

❄ SUITABLE FOR FREEZING

1 Mix together all the ingredients until well combined.
2 Roll into 6–8 balls and flatten into burger shapes.
3 Grill or fry in a little coconut or olive oil for 15–20 minutes, turning halfway, until both sides are coloured and the burgers are cooked through.

 FASCINATING FACT

Check food labels for hydrogenated fats and partially hydrogenated fats. These man-made fats are added to processed foods to increase shelf life, but are bad news for your brain.

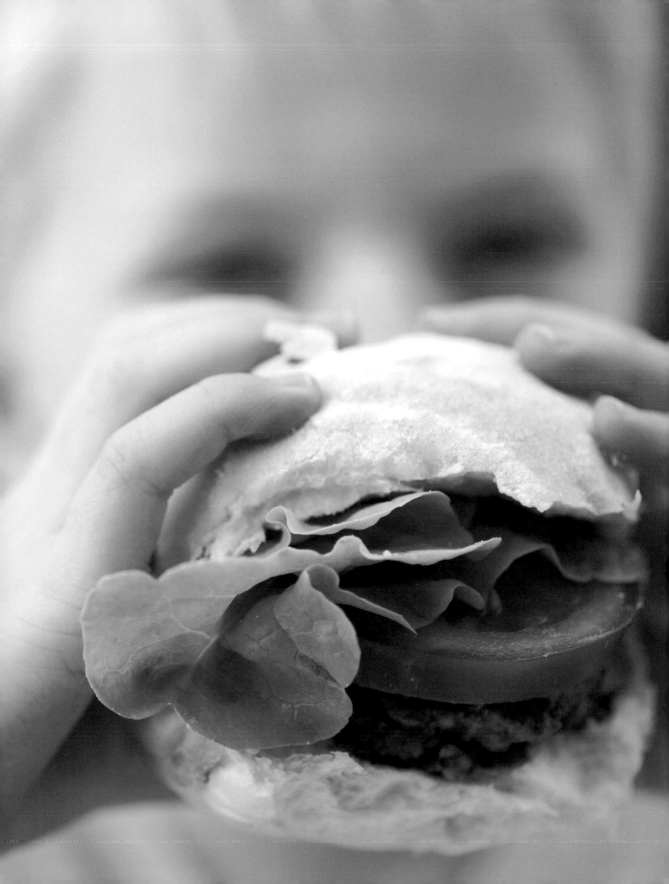

Chicken and Puy Lentil One-Pot Stew

A very easy, one-pot dish that can be made in advance, and is popular with adults and older children. Replace the pepper and leek with carrot and celery, and the lentils with potatoes if you like. This is a complete meal on its own but you can serve it with Sweet Potato Mash (see page 116) to soak up the delicious sauce.

SERVES 4

Parent's verdict: 'Very filling and enjoyable. My youngest (aged 10) wasn't overkeen but the older two loved it.'

2 tbsp olive oil

4 large red onions, peeled and sliced into wedges

4 garlic cloves, crushed

250g (9oz) mushrooms, quartered

2.5cm (1in) piece fresh root ginger, peeled and finely chopped (optional)

3–4 tbsp tomato purée

2 red peppers, deseeded and sliced

2 leeks, sliced

about 4 tsp Marigold Reduced Salt Vegetable Bouillon powder dissolved in 600ml (20fl oz/1 pint) boiling water

200g (7oz) Puy lentils, rinsed

4 large chicken thighs, skinned

freshly ground black pepper

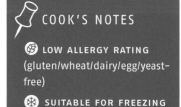

COOK'S NOTES

⊗ **LOW ALLERGY RATING** (gluten/wheat/dairy/egg/yeast-free)

❄ **SUITABLE FOR FREEZING**

1 Heat the oil in a large saucepan or stockpot and add the onions, garlic, mushrooms and ginger, if using. Sauté gently, covered, for 5 minutes, then stir in the tomato purée.

2 Add the remaining ingredients to the pan then cover. Simmer for 35–45 minutes or until the chicken is cooked (check the juices run clear), uncovering halfway through to allow the liquid to reduce and the sauce to thicken. Season with black pepper.

Creamy Cherry Tomato Chicken

This recipe was given to Mrs McDJ by her great friend Jenny and has become a family staple that never fails to please, whether it is served to children or adults. The *crème fraîche* melts into the tomato juices to form a fabulous creamy sauce without too much fat. Serve with baked or mashed potatoes, brown basmati rice or quinoa, plus salad or steamed veg such as broccoli or cauliflower, to help mop up the sauce.

SERVES 4

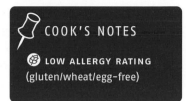

COOK'S NOTES

LOW ALLERGY RATING
(gluten/wheat/egg-free)

2–3 tbsp olive oil

4 chicken breasts, trimmed of fat and skin

450g (1lb) cherry tomatoes

sprinkle of sea salt and freshly ground black pepper

3 tbsp *crème fraîche*

2 tbsp basil leaves, chopped or roughly torn

1 Preheat the oven to 200°C/400°F/Gas 6. Pour the oil into a shallow ovenproof dish (one that can also go on the hob – or use a roasting tin) and add the chicken breasts, turning to coat in the oil.

2 Place the whole cherry tomatoes around the chicken in the dish, season with a little salt and pepper, then cook in the oven for about 50–60 minutes, or until the chicken is done, basting occasionally.

3 Place the dish on the hob and add the *crème fraîche*. Heat gently until it starts to bubble, then simmer for 1–2 minutes, stirring, until the sauce thickens slightly.

4 Stir in the basil just before serving.

Chicken and Vegetable Kebabs

These kebabs are very quick to make and cook, and they particularly appeal to children who like finger food. They can also be barbecued. You will need skewers for this recipe – metal ones are the easiest to use as they don't need soaking, but if you are using wooden ones, soak them in water for 30 minutes before using, to prevent them from burning. Serve with coleslaw, salad and Sweet Potato Wedges (see page 116), Mini Roasties (see page 117), brown basmati rice or quinoa.

SERVES 4

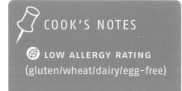

COOK'S NOTES

ⓐ LOW ALLERGY RATING
(gluten/wheat/dairy/egg-free)

> 4 skinless, boneless chicken breasts, cubed
>
> 2 red, yellow or orange peppers, cut into chunks (the same size as the chicken)
>
> 2 courgettes, cut into chunks (the same size as the chicken)
>
> 2 tbsp olive oil
>
> seasoning: either 1 tbsp dried fajita spices or Mediterranean mixed dried herbs, or 1 crushed garlic clove, or simply a sprinkle of sea salt and freshly ground black pepper

1 If using wooden skewers, soak them in water for 30 minutes.
2 Place all the ingredients in a bowl and mix to coat the chicken and vegetables in the oil and seasoning.
3 Preheat the grill to medium.
4 Thread the chicken and vegetables onto skewers or metal kebab sticks, alternating evenly. If you have any leftover pepper pieces, simply add them to the salad or give to your child to nibble on while they are waiting for their meal. Courgette can also be eaten raw, although it has rather too 'earthy' a taste for most children.
5 Grill for 10–15 minutes, turning occasionally until the chicken is cooked through (cut a piece of chicken in half to check that there is no pink meat) and the vegetables are *al dente*, or a bit crunchy to the bite.

Chicken and Vegetable Steam-fry

Steam-frying is just as quick as stir-frying but the food retains more nutrients, as it is steamed rather than being frazzled at very high temperatures. It is a brilliant way to get a variety of vegetables into your child all in one go. You can vary the veg used or, if you are short of time, buy pre-prepared bags of stir-fry vegetables from supermarkets. You can also use turkey, beef strips or tofu instead of chicken. Serve with brown basmati rice, noodles or quinoa.

SERVES 4

1 tbsp coconut oil or olive oil, plus a little extra

4 skinless, boneless chicken breasts, cut into bite-sized pieces

2 garlic cloves, crushed (optional, if time)

2 tsp grated fresh root ginger (optional, if time)

2 red, yellow or orange peppers, thinly sliced

2 carrots, julienne (cut into matchsticks)

4 handfuls mangetouts or sugar snap peas

1 bunch spring onions (about 8), finely sliced on the diagonal

2 tbsp tamari (wheat-free soy sauce), or soy sauce

1 If you don't have a lid with your wok or pan, soak 2 sheets of kitchen paper in cold water and set to one side.

2 Heat 1 tbsp oil in a wok, or large frying pan, and tip to coat the base.

3 Add the meat and stir-fry for 3–5 minutes, or until light brown and cooked through (do this in two batches to avoid over-crowding the pan). Remove from the pan and set to one side.

4 Add a little extra oil to the pan and add the garlic, ginger and vegetables. Stir-fry for 1 minute or so, then add the soy sauce. Stir and cover with a lid or place the damp kitchen paper over the top of the vegetables for a few minutes to allow them to steam underneath.

5 Return the chicken to the pan and stir together; the vegetables should be *al dente*.

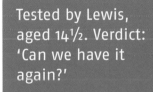

Parent's verdict: 'All the family loved it; lovely and healthy and wholesome as well as being very tasty.'

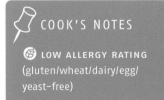

Tested by Lewis, aged 14½. Verdict: 'Can we have it again?'

📌 COOK'S NOTES

🅢 **LOW ALLERGY RATING** (gluten/wheat/dairy/egg/yeast-free)

Chicken Nuggets

We are particularly proud of this recipe – children adore chicken nuggets but they usually feature reconstituted meat and fried, artificially coloured coatings. Our version uses lean chicken goujons dipped in gluten-free, fat-free polenta batter that is then baked, not fried. The result is a golden, just-crisp coating that will help wean any child off frozen or fast-food nuggets and back on to real food. You can dip the whole chicken breast in the mixture to save time slicing and dipping. Serve with Sweet Potato Wedges (see page 116), baked beans and cherry tomatoes.

SERVES 4

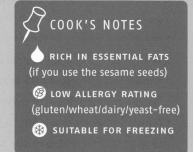

Parent's verdict: 'They loved these – better than McDonalds!'

4 skinless, boneless chicken breasts, sliced into strips (about 4 strips each)

FOR THE BATTER

200g (7oz) instant (pre-cooked) polenta flour

210ml (7fl oz) water

4 eggs, beaten

2 tsp onion salt (or sea salt)

4 tbsp sesame seeds (optional)

COOK'S NOTES

💧 **RICH IN ESSENTIAL FATS** (if you use the sesame seeds)

⊛ **LOW ALLERGY RATING** (gluten/wheat/dairy/yeast-free)

❄ **SUITABLE FOR FREEZING**

1 Preheat the oven to 200°C/400°F/Gas 6. Line a baking tray with greaseproof paper (the batter tends to stick to an oiled tin).

2 Mix together all the batter ingredients in a bowl until smooth. Drop the chicken pieces (one at a time) into the batter and turn over to coat evenly. Place on the baking tray and cook for 15 minutes, or until the meat is cooked through (cut a piece in half and check that the flesh and juices are not pink).

Fajitas

Children adore meals that positively encourage them to play with their food, and fajitas are no exception. Put plates of warmed tortilla wraps on the table with bowls of salsa or cherry tomatoes and sliced spring onions, guacamole or avocado slices and lettuce, as well as this spicy chicken and pepper mixture, and let them create their own fajitas. For a milder version for less adventurous taste buds, omit the fajita spices and season the cooked chicken with a little salt and pepper instead. Make this vegetarian by substituting two large cans of kidney beans for the chicken, and stir into the cooked vegetables. (The fajita seasoning is a dried spice that is available in packets from supermarkets.)

SERVES 4

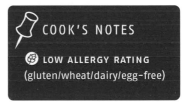

Parent's verdict: 'Joe ate peppers for the first time and loved them – what a bonus.'

COOK'S NOTES

⊛ LOW ALLERGY RATING
(gluten/wheat/dairy/egg-free)

- 4 red onions, sliced
- 2 garlic cloves, crushed
- 4 peppers (choose a mixture of colours), deseeded and sliced lengthways into strips
- 1 tbsp coconut oil or olive oil
- 1½ tbsp fajita seasoning
- 4 chicken breasts, skinned and cut into slices, or 2 × 410g (14½oz) cans kidney beans, drained and rinsed
- 8 corn tortilla wraps (make sure they are gluten-free, if necessary)

1 Sauté or steam-fry the onions, garlic and peppers in the oil for about 5 minutes, or until fairly soft.

2 For chicken fajitas, rub the seasoning into the chicken and grill until cooked (cut a piece in half and check that the juices and flesh are not pink), then stir into the vegetables. For bean fajitas, add the fajita seasoning to the vegetables when cooking, then stir in the drained and rinsed beans, and remove from the heat.

3 Warm the tortilla wraps in a gentle oven or microwave, or according to the packet instructions. Cover to keep warm while on the table.

FISH

A long-acknowledged brain food, fish is an incredibly nutritious choice for children. The omega-3 fats in oily fish – salmon, trout, mackerel, fresh tuna (not canned, as this is stripped of its oils in the canning process), anchovies, sardines, herrings and kippers – cannot be made by the body, so it is essential that we consume them through our diet.

These omega-3 fats are particularly important for children's eye and brain development. In the brain, they help regulate the release and performance of neurotransmitters – the messengers that send information whizzing around. We recommend your family eats oily fish two to three times a week. Other fish types, like haddock, are also healthy choices as they are an excellent source of lean protein, which the brain turns into neurotransmitters.

Easier said than done, you might think, as fish is a notoriously difficult food to persuade children to eat. Lots of children feel squeamish about any fish that doesn't come battered or breadcrumbed, so we have paid particular attention to presenting these recipes in the most palatable, child-friendly format to make sure they get their seal of approval – no fish eyes, tails or bones in sight. The Fish Fingers, for example have a golden polenta-crumb coating for Captain Birds Eye appeal, whereas the Salmon Teriyaki serves bite-sized chunks of skinless, boneless salmon in a sweet soy sauce.

Fish Fingers

Fiona tested this recipe on her parents, who, quite sensibly, think normal fish fingers are revolting, and even they thought these home-made ones were absolutely delicious! Like the Chicken Nuggets (on page 98) the coating is a gluten-free, baked polenta crust that has the same golden, crispy appeal but no fat or additives. We have included optional turmeric in the ingredients if you want to give the coating a more lurid colour akin to frozen ones. Buy undyed haddock to avoid the artificial colours used to turn the dyed smoked haddock bright yellow, or use unsmoked haddock, which is less salty, or any other firm-fleshed fish. Serve with Sweet Potato Wedges (see page 116), Big Baked Beans (see page 111) or canned baked beans and broccoli or peas.

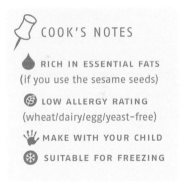

Parent's verdict:
'The kids loved them.'

COOK'S NOTES

● RICH IN ESSENTIAL FATS
(if you use the sesame seeds)

◉ LOW ALLERGY RATING
(wheat/dairy/egg/yeast-free)

✌ MAKE WITH YOUR CHILD

❋ SUITABLE FOR FREEZING

400g (14oz) skinned, undyed, smoked haddock fillet, cut into strips or 'fingers'

FOR THE BATTER
200g (7oz) instant (pre-cooked) polenta flour

210ml (7fl oz) water

4 eggs, beaten

2 tsp onion salt, or sea salt (or 1½ tsp if using smoked haddock, as it is already quite salty)

4 tbsp sesame seeds (optional)

2 tsp ground turmeric (optional)

1 Preheat the oven to 200°C/400°F/Gas 6. Line a baking tray with greaseproof paper (the batter tends to stick to an oiled tin).

2 Mix together all the batter ingredients in a bowl until smooth. Drop the fish fingers, one at a time, into the batter and spoon the mixture over the fish to coat evenly. Place on the baking tray and cook for 10 minutes, so that the coating is crisp and golden and the fish flakes easily.

Tuna and Fresh Tomato Pasta Sauce

A deliciously fresh tomato sauce with a rich, sweet flavour. Cooked tomatoes are an even better source of lycopene (the antioxidant that helps eyesight) than raw ones. This pasta sauce is very cheap and quick to make and goes with almost anything from tuna and pasta to potatoes and chicken or sausages.

SERVES 4

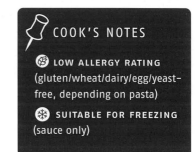

COOK'S NOTES

LOW ALLERGY RATING (gluten/wheat/dairy/egg/yeast-free, depending on pasta)

SUITABLE FOR FREEZING (sauce only)

200g (7oz) wholemeal or gluten/wheat-free pasta

2 × 185g (6½oz) cans (undrained weight) tuna fish in brine or water, or 4 tbsp pine nuts (toasted in a dry frying pan until golden for extra flavour, if time)

FOR THE BASIC TOMATO SAUCE

4 garlic cloves, crushed

2 red onions, finely diced

4 tbsp non-virgin olive oil

2 × 250g (9oz) punnets cherry tomatoes, chopped

4 tbsp tomato purée

sprinkle of sea salt

freshly ground black pepper

1 Cook the pasta according to the packet instructions.
2 Meanwhile, sweat the garlic and onion in the oil in a frying pan for about 3 minutes, or until translucent.
3 Add the tomatoes and cook for 2 minutes, or until they disintegrate.
4 Stir in the tomato purée, reduce the heat and simmer for about 5 minutes, or until rich and thick. Season and taste to check the flavour. You can blend the sauce until smooth to conceal any 'bits' from fusspots, if necessary. Add the cooked pasta to the pan (along with the tuna or pine nuts), stir together and heat through.

Salmon Teriyaki

The sweet flavour of this sauce makes it very popular with children. We suggest cutting the salmon into bite-sized goujons for smaller children, and you could give them chopsticks for an authentic (read: messy and slow) Japanese experience. Salmon is an oily fish, so it provides omega-3 essential brain fats. Serve with brown basmati rice or noodles and Steam-fried Vegetables (see page 118) or steamed vegetables, or add some beansprouts and baby corn, mangetouts or strips of pepper to cook in the salmon parcel. The sauce also works well with chicken goujons (cook at 200°C/400°F/Gas 6 for about 30 minutes).

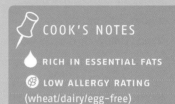

Parent's verdict: 'Really nice, the marinade is great.'

COOK'S NOTES

💧 RICH IN ESSENTIAL FATS

Ⓢ LOW ALLERGY RATING (wheat/dairy/egg-free)

4 skinless, boned salmon fillets, cut into goujons or strips

FOR THE TERIYAKI MARINADE

2 tbsp tamari (wheat-free soy sauce) or soy sauce

2 tbsp mirin (Japanese sweetened rice wine) or water

4 tsp grated fresh root ginger

1 tsp xylitol or caster sugar

1 Mix together all the marinade ingredients. Place the salmon in a bowl and pour the marinade over the top. Stir, then cover and leave for 30 minutes in the fridge if you have time (don't worry if you don't – it will still work but will simply lack the same depth of flavour).
2 While you are waiting for the fish to marinade, preheat the oven to 190°C/375°F/Gas 5. Cut a large square of baking parchment and another of kitchen foil, both large enough to fit the fish inside and to wrap up. Place the baking parchment on top of the foil (this stops the fish from absorbing aluminium from the kitchen foil).
3 Place the salmon in the centre of the baking parchment, pour any remaining marinade over and then fold the foil edges together so that the fish is secured inside a 'parcel'.
4 Place the parcel on a baking tray and cook for 25 minutes.
5 Unwrap the parcel carefully to avoid being burned by the steam, and place the fish on plates. Serve immediately.

Coconut Fish Curry

The sweet, spicy sauce in this curry should appeal to more adventurous palates. It is not overwhelmingly hot and is a good way of sneaking fish into your child's diet. Or, you can replace the fish with 200g (7oz) cooked prawns (add them 2 minutes before the end to heat through). Sneak the onion and pepper past veggie-phobes by finely chopping them (preferably in a food processor) before cooking. Serve with brown basmati rice.

3 tbsp medium curry paste

2 large onions, sliced

2 red, yellow or orange peppers, sliced

1 × 400ml (13½fl oz) can coconut milk (shaken before opening)

300ml (½ pint) hot vegetable stock (or stir 2 tsp Marigold Reduced Salt Vegetable Bouillon powder into 300ml (½ pint) boiling water)

4 firm, skinless white fish fillets (about 600g/1lb 5oz), such as haddock, cut into large chunks (checking for bones with your fingers as you go)

1 Heat the curry paste in a large frying pan or saucepan and fry the onions and peppers for 5 minutes to soften.
2 Pour in the coconut milk and stock, stir and bring to the boil. Reduce the heat and simmer for 5 minutes to thicken slightly, then add the fish and simmer for a further 3–5 minutes, or until the fish flakes easily.

SERVES 4

Parent's verdict: 'We all loved this.'

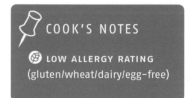

COOK'S NOTES

LOW ALLERGY RATING
(gluten/wheat/dairy/egg-free)

Prawn and Vegetable Steam-fry

Get your child to choose their own vegetables for this steam-fry, then let them help prepare and cook them. If they feel involved and interested in a meal they are more likely to eat it. King prawns have the best texture and flavour but they are more expensive, and normal prawns work fine. Go for organic if you can. Serve with brown basmati rice, noodles or quinoa.

SERVES 4

COOK'S NOTES

⊛ LOW ALLERGY RATING (gluten/wheat/dairy/egg-free)

✋ MAKE WITH YOUR CHILD

1 tbsp coconut oil or olive oil, plus a little extra

2 garlic cloves, crushed (optional, if time)

2 tsp peeled and grated fresh root ginger (optional, if time)

assorted vegetables, such as a bag of beansprouts, 2 finely sliced red, yellow or orange peppers, 2 handfuls of sugar snap peas and 2 handfuls of baby corn

1 bunch spring onions (about 8), finely sliced on the diagonal (optional)

2 tbsp tamari (wheat-free soy sauce) or soy sauce

2 packets (about 400–500g (14oz–1lb 2oz) cooked, peeled prawns

2 tbsp lemon juice

1 If you don't have a lid with your wok or pan, soak 2 sheets of kitchen paper in cold water and set to one side (to be placed over the food in the wok or pan to steam underneath).

2 Heat 1 tbsp oil in a wok or large saucepan and tip to coat the base. Add the garlic and ginger, if using, and the vegetables. Stir-fry for a minute or two then add the tamari or soy sauce. Stir and cover with a lid or place the damp kitchen paper over the top of the vegetables for about 2 minutes to allow them to steam underneath.

3 Add the prawns and lemon juice to the pan and stir-fry for a minute more to warm the prawns through. The vegetables should be *al dente*, or a bit crunchy to the bite.

VEGETARIAN

A vegetarian diet can be a safe and nutritious choice for children if you ensure that it is balanced, with sufficient protein to allow their body to grow and repair itself, and for their brain to make the neurotransmitters required to send and receive information.

Many people get stuck in a cheese rut when catering for vegetarians, but over-reliance on cheese as a source of protein can bring a number of problems. Cheese is high in saturated fat and contributes to inflammatory problems like asthma and eczema. It is also hard to digest and a very common culprit in food allergies, so should not be eaten too often. You can easily get sufficient protein from other foods, such as eggs, nuts and seeds, or by combining beans or lentils with grains to get a full spectrum of the essential amino acids. Quinoa (pronounced 'keenwaa') is a brilliant vegan source of protein, which looks and cooks like couscous and contains just as much protein as animal products, plus plenty of memory-boosting zinc.

These recipes contain lots of interesting and nutritious ingredients to expand your child's diet. Non-vegetarians should also give them a try, as eating a predominantly plant-based diet has been shown to be the healthiest way to eat to avoid disease. Also, several of the recipes in this section can have meat or fish added and so can be adapted for any tastes; see the Egg Fried Rice and the Pitta Pizzas, for example.

We have intentionally restricted the use of green vegetables here, as this seems to be the colour that most children kick up a fuss at. The recipes do still contain plenty of vegetables, but this way you can serve any greens on the side so that the child doesn't spurn the whole dish on the grounds that it has got 'green bits' in it.

Egg Fried Rice

Unfailingly popular with children, including picky eaters, this recipe uses brown basmati rice, which has the least starch of all the rice types, keeping the GL low to make sure blood sugar and energy stay balanced. If your child will eat more vegetables than are used here, by all means add extra (such as onion and mushrooms), but this is a good, nutritious base. Add some toasted cashew nuts instead of egg for vegans, or some diced, cooked ham, chicken, prawns or flaked fish for meat eaters.

SERVES 4

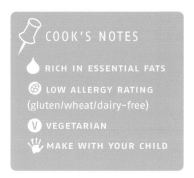

COOK'S NOTES

RICH IN ESSENTIAL FATS

LOW ALLERGY RATING
(gluten/wheat/dairy-free)

V VEGETARIAN

MAKE WITH YOUR CHILD

300g (10½oz) brown basmati rice

1 tbsp coconut oil, olive oil or butter

2 red, yellow or orange peppers, diced

4 free range or organic eggs

200g (7oz) frozen peas

4 tbsp tamari (wheat-free soy sauce) or soy sauce

1 bunch spring onions (about 8), finely sliced (optional, only if your child will eat 'green bits')

1 Cook the rice following the instructions on the packet, but do not add salt or stock or it will be too salty once the tamari or soy sauce is added. Drain and keep warm once ready.

2 While the rice is cooking, heat the oil in a wok or large frying pan and sweat the pepper for 2 minutes until it starts to soften.

3 Break the eggs into the pan and stir-fry so that they start to scramble, then stir in the peas, tamari or soy sauce, and spring onions, if using. Add the cooked rice, mix it all together and serve immediately.

Pitta Pizzas

Pizza is usually a very fatty option, with oil-rich toppings and a base that is full of refined flour and additives. The pitta bread base used here, however, cuts down on refined wheat and saturated fat and you can put a selection of toppings out on the table to let your child create their own 'designer pizza' that is lower in fat. Sprinkle with a little mozzarella or Cheddar cheese instead of overloading the pizza with cheap, processed cheese as is used on many takeaway or frozen pizzas. Non-vegetarians can also use cooked chicken goujons or prawns, canned tuna flakes or strips of lean, unprocessed ham. You can serve the pizzas with salad on the side – try some of the fun ways to present salad and vegetables in the Vegetables section on page 115.

4 wholemeal pitta breads

about 4 tbsp tomato-based pasta sauce, sun-dried tomato paste, tomato purée or passata, or enough to cover one side of each pitta bread

FOR THE TOPPINGS

have a selection of the following: cherry tomatoes, sliced mushrooms, sliced courgette, diced peppers, pitted black olives, sliced mozzarella, grated Cheddar cheese or Parmesan shavings

plus any of the following optional seasonings: a drizzle of olive oil, a little sea salt and freshly ground black pepper, dried oregano or torn, fresh basil leaves

1 Preheat the oven to 240°C/475°F/Gas 9. Spread the top of each pitta bread with tomato sauce, paste, purée or passata, and then scatter with your chosen toppings and seasonings (except for the basil– add before serving) and cook for 10 minutes.

SERVES 4

Parent's verdict: 'Absolutely delicious, I couldn't make enough of these.'

Tested by Lewis, aged 14½. Verdict: 'Not all pizzas are unhealthy, Mum; you were wrong. Got ya!'

COOK'S NOTES

LOW ALLERGY RATING (dairy-free, if made without cheese/egg-free)

V VEGETARIAN

MAKE WITH YOUR CHILD

Sweet Potato and Butterbean Soup

This filling soup gets its wonderfully creamy, thick consistency from the blended butterbeans rather than adding any flour or cream. Its orange colour shows that it is packed with beta-carotene, a vitamin that helps ward off colds and keeps skin healthy. Serve with a piece of bread or a couple of rough oatcakes.

SERVES 4–6

2 medium-sized sweet potatoes, unpeeled and thinly sliced

2 large carrots, sliced

2 red onions, diced

6 tsp Marigold Reduced Salt Vegetable Bouillon powder

1.1 litres (2 pints) boiling water

2 × 410g (14½oz) cans butterbeans, rinsed and drained

freshly ground black pepper

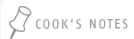

COOK'S NOTES

🌀 LOW ALLERGY RATING (gluten/wheat/dairy/egg/yeast-free)

Ⓥ VEGETARIAN

✋ MAKE WITH YOUR CHILD

❄ SUITABLE FOR FREEZING

1 Place the sweet potatoes, carrots, onions, bouillon powder and water in a large saucepan and bring to the boil. Cover, reduce the heat and simmer for about 20 minutes, or until the sweet potato is cooked (it should be tender and soft when pierced).

2 Add the butterbeans and, using a hand-held blender or a liquidiser, blend until smooth (or leave chunkier if preferred).

3 Sprinkle with plenty of black pepper, taste to check the seasoning, and serve.

Carrot and Lentil Soup

This thick, filling soup has a mild, autumnal flavour that is very popular with children, and by blending the soup you can conceal the onion, celery and lentils – foods which many children would normally turn their noses up at.

SERVES 4
Makes 8 ladlefuls, freeze or refrigerate any leftovers for easy meals

1 tbsp coconut oil, olive oil or butter

2 garlic cloves, crushed

1 onion, roughly chopped

2 large celery sticks, sliced

4 medium–large carrots, sliced

200g (7oz) red split lentils, rinsed

1 litre (just under 2 pints) hot vegetable stock

freshly ground black pepper

1 Heat the oil in a large saucepan and sweat the garlic and onion for 5 minutes to soften.
2 Add the celery, carrots, lentils and stock. Stir and bring to the boil. Cover and simmer for 10 minutes to allow the carrots to soften.
3 Blend, using a hand–held blender or a liquidiser. Season with black pepper and taste – adjust the seasoning if necessary.

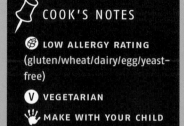

Parent's verdict: 'They loved it!!'

COOK'S NOTES

⊗ LOW ALLERGY RATING (gluten/wheat/dairy/egg/yeast-free)

Ⓥ VEGETARIAN

✋ MAKE WITH YOUR CHILD

❄ SUITABLE FOR FREEZING

Big Baked Beans

One of our greatest success stories – the children make this dish at our Food for the Brain schools' cookery sessions, and by the time they have tasted it they are all converted from the high-sugar, high-salt canned varieties. You can also purée the mixture before adding the beans to make a smooth sauce like the canned versions. Serve on wholemeal or 'all in one' white toast, or toasted rye bread.

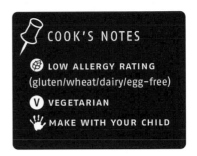

COOK'S NOTES

- LOW ALLERGY RATING (gluten/wheat/dairy/egg-free)
- **V** VEGETARIAN
- MAKE WITH YOUR CHILD

1 tbsp oil

2 red onions, peeled and finely chopped

2 × 410g (14½oz) cans butterbeans, rinsed and drained

2 × 400g (14oz) cans chopped tomatoes

a little salt, or 1 tsp Marigold Reduced Salt Vegetable Bouillon powder

freshly ground black pepper

1 Heat the oil in a saucepan and sauté the onions for 2 minutes to soften.

2 Stir in the remaining ingredients and simmer for 2 minutes, then taste to check the seasoning.

FASCINATING FACT

White flour was first made by flour mills who found that weevils were eating all their grains. The millers removed the husks from the grains, and with them all the goodness, and the weevils left the grains alone – leaving us with a foodstuff so devoid of nutrients that it cannot even support the life of a weevil!

Thick Lentil Stew

Lentils are ridiculously cheap and incredibly nutritious, being packed with fibre, minerals and phytoestrogens to help balance hormones (helpful for children reaching their teens). The lentils soften to form a thick, filling stew that can be used as a sauce with pasta or with a baked potato and salad, or steamed cauliflower or broccoli. Don't worry if you can't get extra vegetables down your child, though, as the stew contains plenty already.

SERVES 4

Parent's verdict: 'Warming and filling. A lovely change from normal stew.'

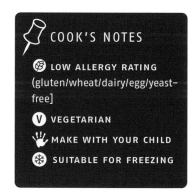

COOK'S NOTES

- ⊗ LOW ALLERGY RATING (gluten/wheat/dairy/egg/yeast-free)
- ⓥ VEGETARIAN
- ✋ MAKE WITH YOUR CHILD
- ❄ SUITABLE FOR FREEZING

1 tsp coconut oil or olive oil

1 garlic clove, crushed

1 onion, chopped

1 pepper, diced

1 small carrot, sliced or grated to hide it

1 celery stick, sliced

125g (just under 5oz) red split lentils, well rinsed and drained

250g punnet cherry tomatoes

1½ tbsp tomato purée

2½ tsp Marigold Reduced Salt Vegetable Bouillon powder, or sea salt to taste

1–2 tsp dried mixed Italian herbs (optional)

freshly ground black pepper

1 Heat the oil in a large frying pan and sweat the garlic, onion, pepper, carrot and celery for about 8 minutes to soften.

2 Add the lentils to the pan and stir well. Cover with cold water and bring to the boil, then boil uncovered for 10 minutes.

3 Add the tomatoes, tomato purée, bouillon powder or salt and herbs, if using, to the pan, cover and reduce the heat. Simmer for 15–20 minutes, or until the stew is thick and the lentils completely soft. If the mixture is too watery, remove the lid to allow some of the liquid to evaporate a few minutes before the end of cooking. Season with black pepper.

Beany Bolognese

A rich bean and tomato stew that can be served with salad or steamed cabbage and pasta or potatoes – top with Sweet Potato Mash (see page 117) to turn it into a nutrient-dense, vegetarian shepherd's pie. It's also packed with fibre and the antioxidant lycopene from the cooked tomatoes.

SERVES 4

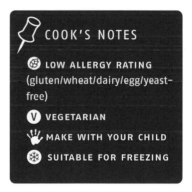

Parent's verdict: 'We all enjoyed this. A great winter warmer.'

2 tsp coconut oil or olive oil

4 garlic cloves, crushed

2 onions, diced

200g (7oz) button mushrooms, cleaned with a brush or wiped with a piece of kitchen paper and sliced

3 tbsp tomato purée

1 × 400g (14oz) can plum tomatoes

2 × 410g (14½oz) cans of borlotti beans, drained and rinsed (or other cooked beans, such as cannellini or haricot)

2 tsp herbes de Provence, or to taste

3 tsp Marigold Reduced Salt Vegetable Bouillon powder, or sea salt to taste

freshly ground black pepper

COOK'S NOTES

⊗ LOW ALLERGY RATING (gluten/wheat/dairy/egg/yeast-free)

Ⓥ VEGETARIAN

✋ MAKE WITH YOUR CHILD

❄ SUITABLE FOR FREEZING

1 Heat the oil and sweat the garlic and onions gently for 2 minutes, then add the mushrooms and cook until fairly soft (about 5 minutes).

2 Add the tomato purée, canned tomatoes, beans and herbs. Add the bouillon powder or salt, and ground black pepper. Simmer for about 5–10 minutes to allow the vegetables to soften and the sauce to thicken. Check the seasoning and adjust if necessary.

Stuffed Peppers

The nuts and mushrooms add a delicious flavour to the rice filling and make this a B-vitamin-rich dish that will help boost mood and energy levels. You can replace the pine nuts with chopped walnuts, or use sunflower or pumpkin seeds. Serve with salad as well if your child will eat it.

4 large red peppers

1 tbsp coconut oil or olive oil

2 medium onions, finely chopped

4 garlic cloves, crushed

300g (10½oz) mushrooms, cleaned with a brush or wiped with a piece of kitchen paper and chopped

2 tsp Marigold Reduced Salt Vegetable Bouillon powder

200g (7oz) brown basmati rice, cooked

2 tbsp pine nuts

handful of fresh basil, chopped (optional)

sea salt and freshly ground black pepper

1 Preheat the oven to 200°C/400°F/Gas 6.
2 Cut the tops off the peppers (reserving the lids), remove the seeds and pith, and slice off the bulbous part inside the pepper that sits below the stalk and contains most of the seeds.
3 Heat the oil in a frying pan and gently sauté the onions and garlic for 2 minutes. Add the mushrooms and bouillon powder, and fry for a further 2–3 minutes.
4 In a large bowl, combine this mixture with the cooked rice, nuts and basil, if using, and season.
5 Stuff the peppers with the mixture and put the tops back on.
6 Place on the baking tray and bake for 35 minutes.

Parent's verdict: 'My husband, John, could eat these all the time, and surprisingly, the children liked them, too – they didn't notice that they contain brown rice'

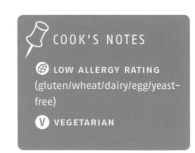

COOK'S NOTES

LOW ALLERGY RATING (gluten/wheat/dairy/egg/yeast-free)

V VEGETARIAN

VEGETABLES

Eating a range of vegetables is a vital part of your child's diet. Vegetables are not only rich in the vitamins and minerals that help fuel brain function, but are also lower in naturally occurring plant sugars than fruit, and are generally richer in the phyto, or plant, nutrients which are so essential for maintaining health and fighting disease.

Ideally try to feed your child vegetables for at least two meals a day. If you are sick of mealtime battles to get your child to eat vegetables, you can sneak them into meals by means of subterfuge: blending onions, peppers and celery into sauces, soups and stews, or grating carrots into Bolognese, for example. These recipes show you plenty of tempting ways to get them to eat their greens . . . and reds, yellows and oranges.

 NEW WAYS WITH VEG

Try these easy and fun ways to present vegetables at mealtimes:

* **Salad on a stick.** Skewer onto cocktail sticks bite-sized chunks of vegetables and fruit, such as cherry tomatoes, cucumber, red, yellow or orange pepper, apple, Satsuma segments or melon chunks.
* **Vegetable sticks** Chop up raw vegetables into bite-sized pieces, or crudités, for your child to nibble on, or dip into hummus, guacamole, cottage cheese or tomato salsa. Go for a rainbow of colours to ensure your child gets a whole range of phyto (plant) nutrients, like red, yellow or orange peppers, celery, cherry tomatoes, baby corn, carrots, cucumber, sugar snap peas, radishes, baby spring onions, even broccoli florets.

Sweet Potato Wedges

These wedges are baked instead of fried, to make them a much healthier alternative to chips. We prefer to use sweet potatoes, as the orange flesh is packed with the antioxidant vitamin beta-carotene, which is very good for the immune system as well as the eyes, but you could use normal potatoes instead.

2 medium–large sweet potatoes, washed but unpeeled, cut into wedges

1 tbsp olive oil

1　Preheat the oven to 180°C/350°F/Gas 4. Place the wedges on a baking tray and drizzle with the oil, shaking to coat.
2　Bake for 40 minutes, turning the wedges halfway through cooking.

> Parent's verdict: 'The sweet potato was too sweet for Paige, but the other two loved them, and I can make it with normal potatoes another time.'

> Tested by Shelley, aged 12. Verdict: 'Loads better than normal chips.'

FASCINATING FACT

Follow the Rainbow Rule when shopping and eating: choose fruits and vegetables in a variety of different colours to ensure that your family eats the whole range of phyto (or plant) nutrients. This is a fun rule for younger children to follow, too; you could even get them to draw a rainbow in black pen, and then colour in a stripe with the appropriate colour after they have eaten a piece of fruit or some vegetables. Photocopy their initial drawing so that you have a new rainbow for them to fill in every day.

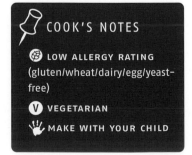

COOK'S NOTES

LOW ALLERGY RATING (gluten/wheat/dairy/egg/yeast-free)

V VEGETARIAN

MAKE WITH YOUR CHILD

116　SMART FOOD FOR SMART KIDS

Sweet Potato Mash

Because they have a naturally creamy flavour, sweet potatoes are ideal for mashing without the need to add extra milk or butter. They also have a beautiful orange colour that not only looks more interesting than normal mash but is also rich in beta-carotene. You can add a sliced carrot to the steamer and mash it with the potato, if you like.

4 medium-sized sweet potatoes (about 450g/1lb), peeled

a little sea salt or about 2 tsp Marigold Reduced Salt Vegetable Bouillon powder

freshly ground black pepper (optional)

1 Slice the sweet potatoes thinly and steam for about 12 minutes, or until soft.
2 Place in a pan and mash roughly, then stir in the seasoning and warm through.

SERVES 4

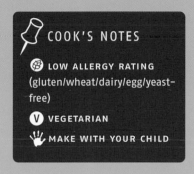

COOK'S NOTES

LOW ALLERGY RATING (gluten/wheat/dairy/egg/yeast-free)

V VEGETARIAN

MAKE WITH YOUR CHILD

Mini Roasties

This is the easiest way to roast potatoes, with no skinning or basting required. The skins become deliciously crisp and retain extra goodness, and the recipe uses far less fat than the traditional method.

700g (1lb 9oz) or about 16 baby new potatoes, rinsed and dried (cut large ones in half so that they are all roughly the same size to cook evenly)

drizzle of non-virgin olive oil

sprinkle of sea salt

1 Preheat the oven to 180°C/350°F/Gas 4. Place the potatoes in a roasting tin and drizzle with a little oil, then sprinkle with sea salt.
2 Shake the tin to coat the potatoes evenly and place in the oven for about 1 hour, taking the tray out and shaking halfway through to turn the potatoes.

SERVES 4

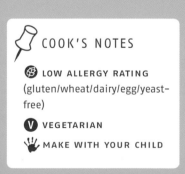

COOK'S NOTES

LOW ALLERGY RATING (gluten/wheat/dairy/egg/yeast-free)

V VEGETARIAN

MAKE WITH YOUR CHILD

Steam-fried Vegetables

Like stir-frying, steam-frying is a brilliant way to get your child to eat all kinds of vegetables. Apply the Rainbow Rule: try to get as many different coloured vegetables on the plate as possible, to ensure a maximum range of nutrients. Or, if they turn their nose up at lots of different veg, find one they like, such as cabbage, for example, which is delicious sprinkled with tamari or soy sauce and toasted sesame seeds.

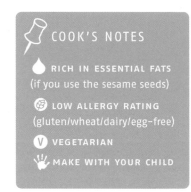

COOK'S NOTES

RICH IN ESSENTIAL FATS
(if you use the sesame seeds)

LOW ALLERGY RATING
(gluten/wheat/dairy/egg-free)

V VEGETARIAN

MAKE WITH YOUR CHILD

1 tbsp coconut oil or olive oil, plus a little extra

2 garlic cloves, crushed (optional, if time)

2 tsp peeled and grated fresh root ginger (optional, if time)

assorted vegetables, such as 2 red, yellow or orange peppers and 2 carrots, finely sliced into strips, and 2 handfuls of mangetouts, sugar snap peas, broccoli florets and/or baby corn

1 bunch spring onions (about 8), finely sliced on the diagonal (optional)

2 tbsp tamari (wheat-free soy sauce) or soy sauce

drizzle of toasted sesame oil, to taste (optional)

2 tbsp sesame seeds, toasted in a dry frying pan until they start to turn golden (optional)

1 If you don't have a lid with your wok or pan, soak 2 sheets of kitchen paper in cold water and set to one side (to be placed over the food in the wok or pan to steam underneath).

2 Heat the oil in a wok or large saucepan and tip to coat the base. Add the garlic and ginger, if using, and the vegetables. Stir-fry for a minute or two then add the tamari or soy sauce. Stir and cover with a lid or place the damp kitchen paper over the top of the vegetables for 2 minutes to allow them to steam underneath. The vegetables should be al dente, or a bit crunchy to the bite. Drizzle with toasted sesame oil and sprinkle with the sesame seeds, if using.

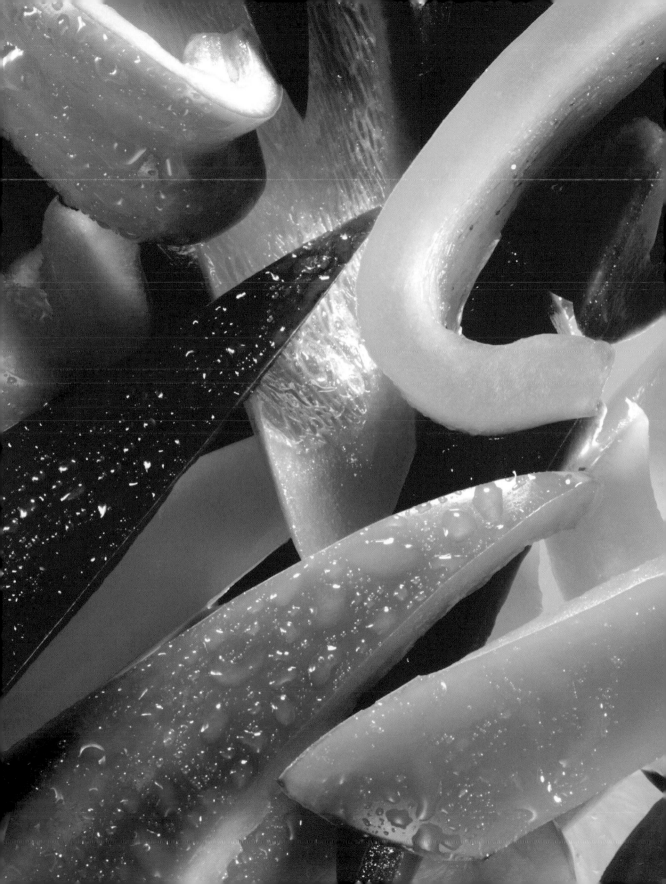

Corn on the Cob

Finger food always appeals to children. Corn on the cob is naturally sweet and juicy, without having the added salt and sugar of most canned sweetcorn. Some people like to add a little salt and butter to the cob, but we think they are delicious as they are. Corn on the cob can also be microwaved on high for 3–5 minutes, or until tender.

SERVES 4

4 corn on the cobs

1 Strip the outer husks from the corn cobs if necessary. Place in a large pan of boiling water (you may need to cook them in two pans) and cook for 5 minutes. Don't add salt to the cooking water or it will toughen the corn.
2 Drain and rinse with cold water, then leave to rest for 1 minute to allow them to cool down before serving.

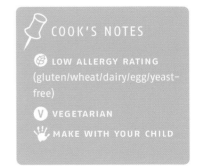

COOK'S NOTES

⊛ LOW ALLERGY RATING (gluten/wheat/dairy/egg/yeast-free)

Ⓥ VEGETARIAN

✋ MAKE WITH YOUR CHILD

Red Pepper and Cucumber Salsa

Zesty without being too hot, this salsa will help to liven up burgers or a simple chicken and salad wrap.

SERVES 2

1 medium-sized red onion, diced

4 cherry tomatoes, cut into small chunks

½ red pepper, diced

1 tbsp extra virgin olive oil

2 tsp finely chopped flat-leaf parsley

5cm (2in) piece of cucumber, cut lengthways into quarters then sliced horizontally into triangles

2 tsp lemon juice

freshly ground black pepper

Mix all of the ingredients together.

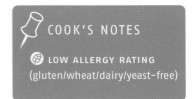

COOK'S NOTES

⊛ LOW ALLERGY RATING (gluten/wheat/dairy/yeast-free)

Guacamole

If you have time you can make this delicious, very refreshing avocado dip and serve it with crudités (vegetable sticks). If your child doesn't like hot or strong flavours, omit the garlic and onion. You can even simply mash an avocado with a little lemon or lime juice for the simplest, mildest version.

SERVES 2

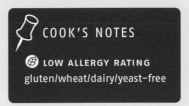

COOK'S NOTES

LOW ALLERGY RATING
gluten/wheat/dairy/yeast-free

1 ripe avocado
juice of ½ lime or ¼ lemon
½ garlic clove, crushed
½ small red onion, finely diced
1 tomato, deseeded and diced
1 tbsp chopped fresh coriander and/or flat-leaf parsley (optional)
1 tbsp extra virgin olive oil
freshly ground black pepper

1 Cut the avocado in half lengthways and remove the stone.
2 Scrape the flesh out of the shell into a bowl and quickly mash with the lime or lemon juice to prevent discolouration. Stir in the remaining ingredients and taste to check the seasoning.

Little Gem Salad Boats

Break off Little Gem lettuce leaves, wash and dry them, then fill with chopped vegetables, such as cherry tomatoes, cucumber, baby corn and peppers, so that they sit like a boat on the plate and can be picked up and eaten with the fingers. You can also add a spoonful of hummus, guacamole, cottage cheese, tomato salsa, or tuna or egg mayonnaise to the base of the boat, and sprinkle cress or alfalfa sprouts on top.

Puddings

Most of the recipes in this chapter feature fruit and whole-grains, to help you increase your child's intake without a struggle. They are also sugar-free or very low in sugar, and are sweetened instead with fruit or with xylitol, the only sugar alternative that we recommend. This near-miraculous ingredient doesn't upset blood sugar levels, unlike other sweeteners, including normal sugar, fructose, artificial sweeteners, dried fruit, syrup or honey. In fact, you would have to eat nine spoons of xylitol to have the same effect on your blood sugar as one spoon of sugar! It also doesn't have an unpleasant chemical aftertaste like so many artificial alternatives, as it is a naturally occurring substance found in many plants. See the Resources section for suppliers.

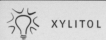 XYLITOL

We use xylitol in several recipes in this chapter. When first using xylitol, increase your daily intake gradually to allow the body to adjust, as large quantities can have a laxative effect. Don't let your child go berserk sweetening their cereal, puddings or drinks with xylitol – they may get a runny tummy as a result. Used in moderation it is a healthy way to include sweet treats in your diet. Do not give to very young children (under two), however, as it is important to get high-calorie, nutrient-dense foods into them as their stomachs are small.

Plum Crumble

Fiona's all-time favourite pudding, and a recipe she is particularly proud of, as the topping is every bit as delicious as a standard wheat, butter and sugar-based crumble, but it is low GL and wheat-free. Serve on its own or with custard (made with xylitol instead of sugar), live natural yoghurt or a little vanilla ice cream.

SERVES 6

FOR THE CRUMBLE

150g (5½oz) whole oatflakes

65g (2¼oz) coconut oil or butter, at room temperature

75g (3oz) xylitol

75g (3oz) ground almonds

FOR THE FILLING

900g (2lb) plums, halved and stoned

1 tsp ground cinnamon

100g (3½oz) xylitol

1 Preheat the oven to 180°C/350°F/Gas 4. Whizz the oats in a food processor, nut mill or coffee grinder to grind into flour. Add the coconut oil or butter and whizz again to form crumbs. Mix in the xylitol and ground almonds.

2 Place the plum halves in the base of a large, shallow ovenproof dish, sprinkle with the cinnamon and xylitol then top with the crumble mixture. Even out the top, then bake for 30–40 minutes, or until the top starts to turn golden brown and the plum juice is bubbling.

Tested by Carl and Tom, aged 13. Verdict: 'As squidgy and sweet as normal crumble'

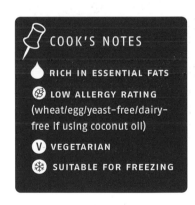

COOK'S NOTES

RICH IN ESSENTIAL FATS

LOW ALLERGY RATING (wheat/egg/yeast-free/dairy-free if using coconut oil)

V VEGETARIAN

SUITABLE FOR FREEZING

Apple Cobbler

This is a proper, seriously filling British pudding. The apple-pie-style dish has a gluten-free topping made of cornmeal and ground almonds, so it is much easier to digest and has a lower GL than pastry. The cinnamon not only adds flavour but it also helps the body balance blood sugar.

Parent's verdict: 'Very tasty.'

Children's verdict: 'Really filling and tastes great.'

FOR THE APPLE FILLING

3 Bramley (cooking) apples, cored and roughly chopped (unpeeled – the peel softens completely upon cooking)

1½ tsp ground cinnamon

1½ tbsp lemon juice or water

1½ tbsp xylitol

FOR THE TOPPING

75g (3oz) cornmeal or instant (pre-cooked) polenta flour

75g (3oz) ground almonds

100g (3½oz) xylitol

½ tsp ground cinnamon

2 tsp coconut oil or butter

75ml (2½fl oz) milk or non-dairy milk

1 medium-sized free range egg, lightly beaten

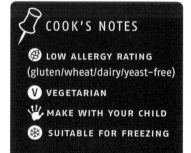

COOK'S NOTES

 LOW ALLERGY RATING (gluten/wheat/dairy/yeast-free)

V VEGETARIAN

 MAKE WITH YOUR CHILD

 SUITABLE FOR FREEZING

1 Preheat the oven to 200°C/400°F/Gas 6. Place the apple filling ingredients in a pan and gently stew for around 5 minutes until fairly soft. Add extra water if the pan dries up. Spoon into an ovenproof dish.

2 Mix the cornmeal or polenta flour, ground almonds, xylitol and cinnamon together in a mixing bowl.

3 Gently melt the coconut oil or butter in a pan then stir it into the dry mixture along with the milk and beaten egg.

4 Spoon the topping over the cooked apple and bake for 35 minutes, or until the top is firm to the touch and cooked through (spear with a skewer to make sure the topping isn't still gooey underneath). You may need to cover the top with kitchen foil after 30 minutes or so to prevent it from going too brown.

Fruit Compote with Yoghurt

Take advantage of the glut of British fruit available in the summer and stew them to make delicious, fibre- and vitamin-packed compotes. You can also top with Jolly Healthy Granola (see page 69) for an instant crumble.

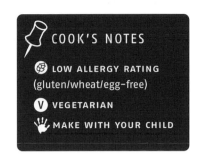

your choice of fruit, such as 3 Bramley (cooking) apples or 4 pears, or 8 plums or apricots, cored and stoned, if necessary, then roughly chopped

1–2 tbsp water

xylitol, to taste (depending on the sweetness of the fruit you use)

ground cinnamon or ginger, to taste (optional)

300g (10½oz) live natural yoghurt

1 Place the fruit in a saucepan and add a splash of water, then simmer gently for about 5 minutes, or until the fruit softens.

2 Sweeten to taste with xylitol. Add a little ground ginger or cinnamon for added flavour, if you like. Serve with the yoghurt.

Instant Frozen Yogurt

This fabulously delicious pudding is just as good as ice cream but low in fat, sugar-free, bursting with vitamin C and can be made in minutes – no need to freeze in advance or churn every four hours.

SERVES 4

400g (14oz) frozen mixed berries (available in bags from supermarkets; leave them to defrost for a few minutes first if your blender won't cope with fully frozen ones)

400g (14oz) live natural yoghurt

4 tbsp xylitol, or to taste

Blend everything together until smooth and the consistency of sorbet or frozen yoghurt. Eat quickly before it melts (if it does melt it makes a scrummy drink, though).

Parent's verdict: 'Thought they were going to lick the bowls out.'

Tested on Paige, aged 10. Verdict: 'Best thing in the world, next bowl, please.'

> ⛯ **FASCINATING FACT**
>
> A pot of fruit yoghurt can contain as much as six teaspoons of sugar! Blend or chop fresh fruit and stir into live natural yoghurt for a fresh, sugar-free alternative with much more flavour.

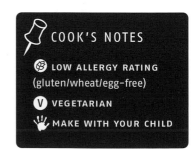

📌 **COOK'S NOTES**

🍇 LOW ALLERGY RATING (gluten/wheat/egg-free)

Ⓥ VEGETARIAN

🖐 MAKE WITH YOUR CHILD

Chocolate Orange Mousse

A seriously good pud, and worthy of serving at a dinner party as well as to children. The addition of orange juice ensures the mousse is not too rich, and the lack of butter and cream cuts down on unnecessary fat and dairy products. Dark chocolate is richer in cocoa solids and lower in sugar than cheap milk chocolate, so you need less of it for the same effect. For a serious pudding blowout, try it with strawberries and the Banana Cheesecake (on page 130). The flavour improves if the mousse is made a day in advance.

SERVES 4

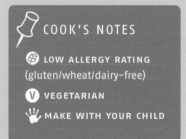

Parent's verdict: 'Brilliant – we all thoroughly enjoyed it'

180g (just over 6oz) good-quality dark chocolate (check it is dairy-free, if necessary), broken into pieces

150ml (¼ pt) freshly squeezed or pure (no added sugar) orange juice

6 medium-sized free range or organic eggs, separated

1 Melt the chocolate over a *bain-marie* (place the chocolate in a heatproof bowl over a pan of simmering water, taking care not to let the water touch the base of the bowl), stirring as the mixture thickens to a thick cream. Alternatively melt the chocolate in a microwave.

2 Add the juice to the bowl and cook with the chocolate over a gentle heat until it forms a creamy consistency. This takes quite a long time and the mixture won't get very thick, but it should be fairly gloopy and move slowly when running over the back of a spoon.

3 Remove from the heat and beat in the egg yolks, one at a time.

4 Beat the egg whites until they form stiff peaks, then gently fold a spoonful of the beaten egg into the chocolate mixture to loosen it, carefully using a metal spoon so that you don't knock out all the air. Fold in the remaining egg and carefully spoon the mousse into a large bowl and place immediately in the fridge to set (this will take at least 1 hour).

COOK'S NOTES

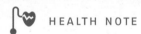

LOW ALLERGY RATING (gluten/wheat/dairy-free)

V VEGETARIAN

MAKE WITH YOUR CHILD

HEALTH NOTE

Because this recipe contains raw egg, always choose organic, or at the very least free range, eggs to reduce the likelihood of salmonella contamination, and do not serve to pregnant women, very young children, the elderly or infirm.

Banana Cheesecake

Another fabulous cheesecake that has a wheat-free base using oatcakes and chopped nuts. To make this nut-free, replace the nuts with an extra 100g (3½oz) of oatcakes. The filling contains a little tahini, which blends with the banana and xylitol to give a slightly fudgey, or banoffee-ish flavour. Absolutely delicious with chopped strawberries.

SERVES 8–10

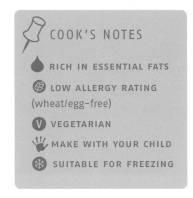

COOK'S NOTES

● RICH IN ESSENTIAL FATS

⊗ LOW ALLERGY RATING (wheat/egg-free)

Ⓥ VEGETARIAN

🖐 MAKE WITH YOUR CHILD

❄ SUITABLE FOR FREEZING

FOR THE BASE

100g (3½oz) rough oatcakes

100g (3½oz) unsalted nuts and/or seeds (hazelnuts, almonds, walnuts, brazil nuts and sunflower seeds all work well)

50g (2oz) coconut oil or butter

30g (just over 1oz) xylitol

FOR THE FILLING

375g (13oz) plain cottage cheese

300g (10½oz) natural yoghurt

3 tbsp tahini

about 75g (3oz) xylitol

3 bananas

1 Preheat the oven to 160°C/325°F/Gas 3. Line a 20cm (8in) loose-based cake tin with baking parchment.

2 Place the ingredients for the base in a food processor and whizz until the consistency of coarse breadcrumbs. (Alternatively, grind the nuts and oatcakes in a nut mill or coffee grinder then transfer to a bowl.) Stir in the oil or butter and xylitol. Press firmly into the base of the lined cake tin using the underside of a metal tablespoon, so that it covers the base evenly. Bake for 10 minutes then set aside to cool.

3 Meanwhile, blend the filling ingredients in a food processor or using a blender until smooth. Taste and add a little more xylitol to sweeten, if necessary. Pour into the cake tin and cook for about 1 hour, or until the top is just firm to the touch. Allow to cool on a wire rack, then chill.

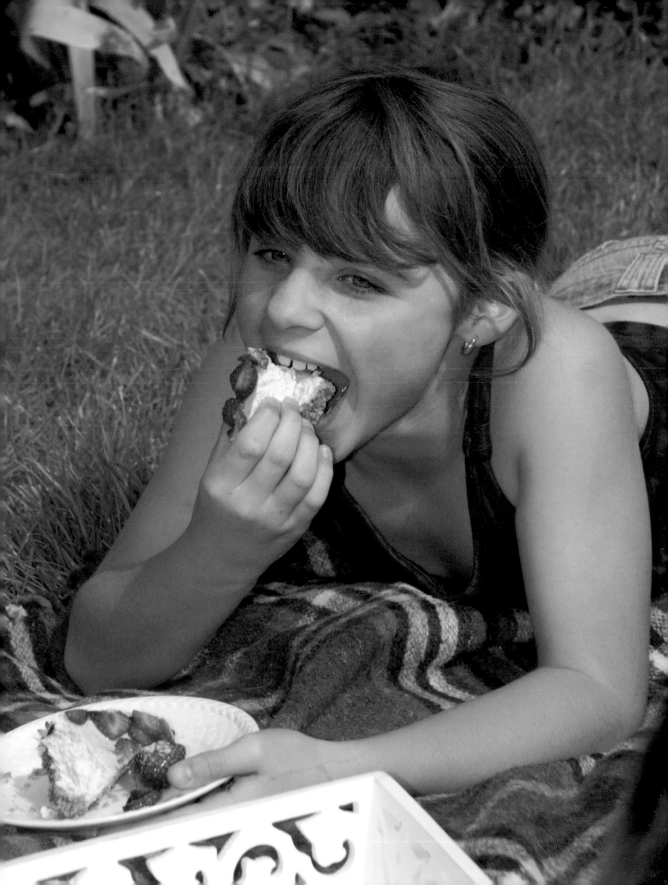

Chocolate Cheesecake

If you want a pudding with the wow factor, serve this with some chopped strawberries. To make a nut-free base, replace the nuts with an extra 100g (3½oz) of oatcakes.

Tested by: Tom, aged 13. Verdict: 'Yummy!'

FOR THE BASE

100g (3½oz) unsalted nuts and/or seeds (hazelnuts, almonds, walnuts, brazil nuts and sunflower seeds all work well)

100g (3½oz) rough oatcakes

50g (2oz) coconut oil or butter

30g (just over 1oz) xylitol

FOR THE FILLING

400g (14oz) dark chocolate, broken into chunks

375g (13oz) plain cottage cheese

300g (10½oz) natural yoghurt

2 free range egg yolks

4 free range egg whites (use up the leftover yolks in the Marzipan Shapes on page 141)

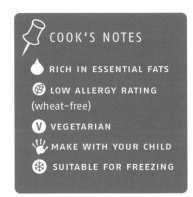

COOK'S NOTES

○ RICH IN ESSENTIAL FATS

✪ LOW ALLERGY RATING (wheat-free)

Ⓥ VEGETARIAN

🖐 MAKE WITH YOUR CHILD

❄ SUITABLE FOR FREEZING

1 Preheat the oven to 160°C/325°F/Gas 3. Line a 20cm (8in) loose-based cake tin with baking parchment.

2 Place the ingredients for the base in a food processor and whizz until the consistency of coarse breadcrumbs (or alternatively, grind the nuts and oatcakes then transfer to a bowl. Stir in the oil or butter and xylitol.) Press firmly into the bottom of the lined cake tin using the underside of a metal tablespoon, so that it covers the base evenly. Bake for 10 minutes then set aside.

3 Meanwhile, melt the chocolate over a *bain-marie* or in a microwave.

4 Blend the cottage cheese, yoghurt and melted chocolate until smooth, then quickly blend in the egg yolks.

5 Beat the egg whites until they form stiff peaks, then gently fold them into the chocolate mixture until evenly blended. Pour into the cake tin and cook for about 1–1¼ hours, or until the top is just firm to the touch. Allow to cool on a wire rack, then chill.

Parties

There is absolutely no need to turn your child into a social pariah by banishing cakes and sweet things when they have friends round for tea. There are plenty of cakes, biscuits and home-made sweets that taste delicious but still follow the healthy eating guidelines we recommend throughout this book (see the Cakes, Biscuits and Sweets section on page 133).

If you are throwing a children's party, here are some tips to help avoid your child and their friends turning into hyperactive horrors:

* Serve savoury foods first so that they don't fill up on sweets.
* Avoid free-for-all buffets – they may seem like less work, but, given a free rein, some children will eat chocolate biscuits exclusively.
* Serve our delicious drinks, such as our home-made Lemonade or Strawberry Fizz (both page 143) instead of additive-ridden soft drinks.

Savoury nibbles

Our experience shows that children almost always reject sandwiches at parties, perhaps because many are faced with them every day in packed lunches. The parents we have spoken to all agree, however, that providing lots of savoury items before you bring out the cakes and biscuits definitely helps to fill the children up so that they eat less sugary stuff. We have therefore come up with some more interesting snacks and dishes:

* **Seasoned, toasted nuts and seeds** (see page 80).
* **Crudités** (chopped vegetable sticks) with hummus, cream cheese, guacamole (either bought or home-made – see recipe on page 121) or salsa (bought or home made – see recipe on page 120).
* **Mini oatcakes** with Marmite and cress, or cream cheese and ham, or hummus, guacamole (again either bought or see recipe on page 121) or salsa (bought or see recipe on page 120).
* **Watermelon and feta cubes** on cocktail sticks.
* **Bite-sized fruit chunks** Serve easy-to-eat, finger-food fruit such as grapes, satsuma segments, apple and banana chunks – drizzled with a little lemon juice to stop them going brown.
* **Pitta Pizzas**, cut into bite-sized pieces (see page 108).
* **Chicken and Vegetable Kebabs** (see page 96).
* **Mini Roasties** (see page 117) sprinkled with grated cheese.
* **Burgers** (see page 92) – make these into much smaller, mini burgers for finger food, or stuff into pitta bread with salad.
* **Mini sandwiches on wholemeal/'all-in-one' white bread** (see the ideas on page 84).

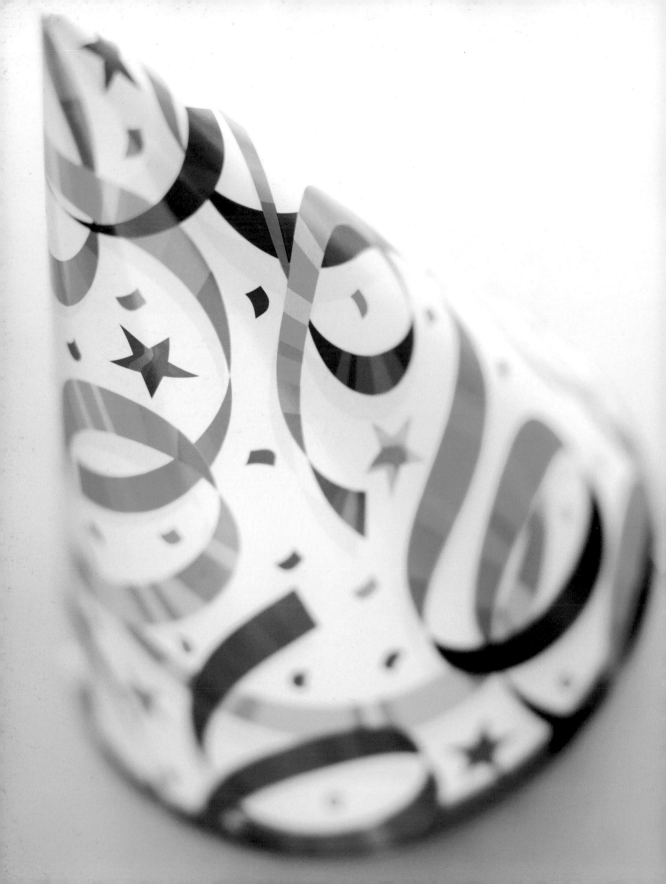

Cakes, Biscuits and Sweets

Our cakes, biscuits and sweets make useful additions to lunch boxes, and no self-respecting party is complete without sticky cakes and biscuits. There is no reason why your child should forego sweet treats just because they are eating healthily. By using wholegrains, nuts and seeds you can keep the GL of the dish low and avoid the digestive and allergy problems associated with refined wheat-flour products. Fruit and wholegrains are used where possible, and the natural sugar alternative, xylitol, that has the same sweet taste as sugar but doesn't upset blood sugar levels, replaces sugar for a sweet taste without the sugar rush.

 XYLITOL

When first using xylitol, increase your daily intake gradually to allow the body to adjust, as large quantities can have a laxative effect. Don't let your child go berserk sweetening their cereal, puddings or drinks with xylitol – they may get a runny tummy as a result. Used in moderation it is a healthy way to include sweet treats in your diet. Do not give to very young children (under two), however, as it is important to get high-calorie, nutrient-dense foods into them as their stomachs are small.

Chocolate Cake with Cream Cheese Frosting

Heaven knows who thought up the combination of chocolate and courgette, but this rich, gooey cake is absolutely delicious, and has been a great favourite with all the children we have tested it on. If your child baulks at the idea of green vegetables, just don't mention the courgette, because once this is cooked with the chocolate they simply won't notice it. Store in an airtight container in the fridge on account of the cream cheese frosting.

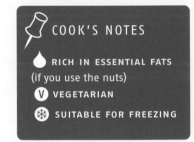

Children's verdict: 'Yummy, yummy in our tummies – more, please.'

200g (7oz) plain flour

½ tsp bicarbonate of soda

1 tsp baking powder

½ tsp salt

100g (3½oz) xylitol

2 medium-sized free range or organic eggs

180ml (6fl oz) olive oil

170g (just under 6oz) good-quality dark chocolate

225g (8oz) courgettes, grated

55g (just over 2oz) walnuts or hazelnuts, finely chopped (optional)

FOR THE CREAM CHEESE FROSTING

about 250g (9oz) low-fat cream cheese

½ tsp vanilla extract

1 tbsp xylitol

COOK'S NOTES

RICH IN ESSENTIAL FATS (if you use the nuts)

V VEGETARIAN

SUITABLE FOR FREEZING

1 Preheat the oven to 180°C/350°F/Gas 4. Line the base of a 20cm (8in) loose-based cake tin with baking parchment and grease the sides.
2 Sift the flour, bicarbonate of soda, baking powder and salt into a bowl. Stir in the xylitol.
3 In a separate bowl, beat the eggs into the oil.
4 Melt the chocolate over a bain marie (place the chocolate in a heatproof bowl over a pan of simmering water, taking

care not to let the water touch the base of the bowl) or in a microwave.

5 Stir the eggs and oil into the dry ingredients then mix in the melted chocolate, courgettes and nuts, if using.

6 Pour the mixture into the prepared cake tin and bake for 25–30 minutes, or until the cake is well risen and firm to the touch, and an inserted skewer comes out clean. Allow to cool on a wire rack before icing.

7 To make the cream cheese frosting, mix together the cream cheese, vanilla extract and xylitol until smooth, then spread on the cake (though if freezing, don't ice the cake until after it has defrosted).

Coconut Snowball Biscuits

Soft, lemony coconut balls that are very easy for children to make. They are also gluten-, dairy- and sugar-free.

MAKES 10
(SERVES ABOUT 3)

140g (5oz) desiccated coconut

3 egg whites

3 tbsp xylitol

1½ tbsp lemon juice

1 tbsp cornflour

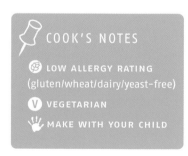

COOK'S NOTES

LOW ALLERGY RATING
(gluten/wheat/dairy/yeast-free)

V VEGETARIAN

MAKE WITH YOUR CHILD

1 Preheat the oven to 180°C/350°F/Gas 4. Line a large baking tray with baking parchment.

2 Combine all the ingredients in a mixing bowl to form a paste.

3 Shape into ten balls using your hands (press quite firmly to make sure they don't fall apart after cooking). Bake for 20 minutes, then leave to cool before storing in an airtight container.

Apple and Almond Tray Bake

This delicious, moist cake can be enjoyed with a clean conscience, as it has a very low GL and contains no wheat or flour, sugar or fat and is packed with protein, calcium and fibre. It makes a nutritious snack or lunch-box treat, or can be served warm with custard (made with xylitol instead of sugar) for pudding.

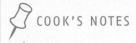

COOK'S NOTES

◆ RICH IN ESSENTIAL FATS

Ⓖ LOW ALLERGY RATING
(gluten/wheat/dairy/yeast-free)

Ⓥ VEGETARIAN

❄ SUITABLE FOR FREEZING

3 Bramley (cooking) apples, about 550g/1¼lb in total, unpeeled, cored and diced

250g (9oz) ground almonds

2 tsp ground cinnamon

½ tsp baking powder

3 medium-sized free range or organic eggs

150g (5½oz) xylitol

Around 85g (just over 3oz) flaked almonds for sprinkling on top

1 Preheat the oven to 180°C/350°F/Gas 4. Line a baking tin, about 20 × 30cm (8 × 12in), with baking parchment.
2 Place the apples, ground almonds, cinnamon and baking powder in a mixing bowl and stir together. Set to one side.
3 Beat the eggs and xylitol in a clean mixing bowl until they become pale and creamy and start to thicken slightly (the whisk should leave a trail when lifted out of the mixture).
4 Gradually fold the apple and almond mixture into the beaten egg, using a metal tablespoon, and taking care not to knock all of the air out of the egg (this is easiest done by drawing a figure-of-eight shape with the spoon as you fold).
5 Quickly pour the cake mixture into the prepared tin and sprinkle with the flaked almonds. Bake for 45–50 minutes, or until golden and fairly firm to the touch (cover the top with kitchen foil towards the end of cooking to prevent the almonds from scorching, if necessary). Leave to cool on a wire rack before cutting into slices and storing in an airtight container.

Easiest Ever Flapjacks

An ideal recipe for children to make, as it is simply stirred together before cooking. This must be the only flapjack recipe to avoid the usual syrup or honey binders, but which is still finger-lickingly gooey and holds together. The nuts provide protein to lower the GL of the flapjack, as well as minerals and essential fats. You can also add 1–2 teaspoons or so of ground ginger, to taste.

Parent's verdict: 'The children loved them. We did, too.'

150g (5½oz) slightly salted butter or coconut oil (this makes it dairy-free but the flavour is not as good), at room temperature or just above

150g (5½oz) xylitol

150g (5½oz) roughly chopped nuts, such as a mixture of almonds and hazelnuts, or pecan nuts and brazil nuts (or use seeds or replace with oats in cases of nut allergies)

150g (5½oz) whole rolled oats

1 Preheat the oven to 180°C/350°F/Gas 4. Line a baking tin, about 20 × 30cm (8 × 12in) with baking parchment.

2 Beat the butter or coconut oil with the xylitol until it is creamy, then stir in the nuts and oats.

3 Spoon into the prepared tin and bake for 20–25 minutes, or until golden brown (they still won't set until they cool down). Slice into fingers, and allow to cool and harden in the tin set on a wire rack before storing in an airtight container. These can also be frozen – defrost individual flapjacks as and when you need them.

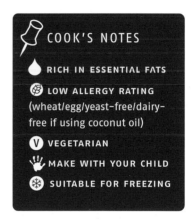

COOK'S NOTES

● RICH IN ESSENTIAL FATS

◉ LOW ALLERGY RATING (wheat/egg/yeast-free/dairy-free if using coconut oil)

Ⓥ VEGETARIAN

🖐 MAKE WITH YOUR CHILD

❄ SUITABLE FOR FREEZING

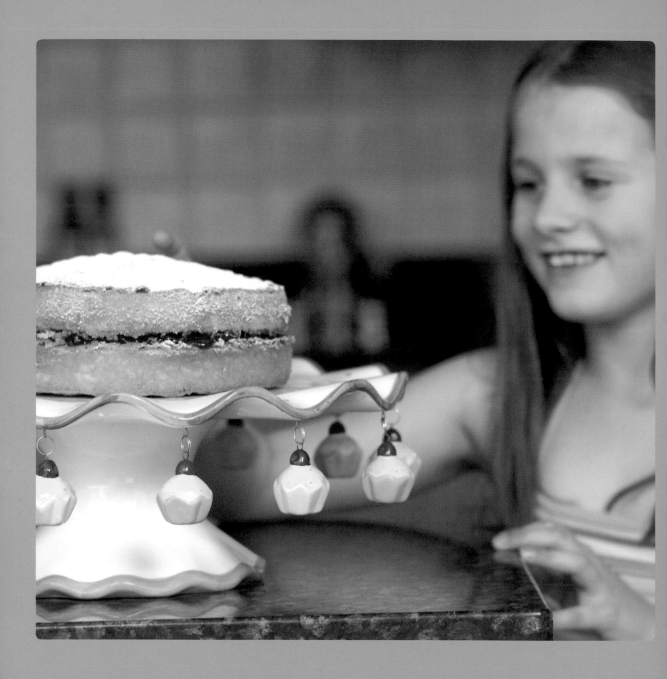

Victoria Sponge with Jam

This foolproof sponge recipe is sugar-free and very light and moist. Plus, the xylitol makes the cake easier to slice without crumbling.

175g (6oz) self-raising flour

1 tsp baking powder

175g (6oz) xylitol

175g (6oz) butter, or half butter and half margarine, at room temperature

3 large free range or organic eggs, at room temperature

3 drops vanilla extract

good-quality sugar-free jam or compote for the filling, such as raspberry or apricot (choose one with a high fruit content and no artificial sweeteners)

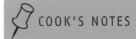

COOK'S NOTES

 VEGETARIAN

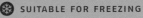 SUITABLE FOR FREEZING

1 Preheat the oven to 160°C/325°F/Gas 3. Grease and line a 20cm (8in) cake tin.
2 Sift the flour and baking powder into a mixing bowl.
3 Add the xylitol, fat, eggs and vanilla, and whisk until the mixture is well combined and creamy (this is easiest done using an electric hand whisk). Test the consistency by taking a teaspoonful of mixture and tapping it on the side of the bowl – it should fall off easily. If it is too thick, whisk 1–2 tsp warm water into the mixture.
4 Spoon the mixture into the prepared cake tin and level off the top. Bake in the centre of the oven for about 45–55 minutes, or until the top is golden and springy to the touch, and a skewer inserted into the middle comes out clean.
5 Leave to cool for a few minutes then loosen the edges with a palette knife and carefully turn the cake out onto a wire cooling rack. Peel off the baking parchment.
6 When the cake is nearly cool, carefully slice the cake into two layers and sandwich together with jam.

Chocolate Crunchies

A seriously delicious but very nutritious take on an old
favourite. Bound together with a little chocolate and nut
butter instead of syrup, they conceal plenty of essential fats,
protein, minerals and vitamins. You can vary the mixture of
oats, nuts and seeds according to what your child will eat,
but this is a fabulous way to conceal superfoods like seeds
within a delicious teatime treat.

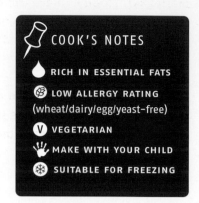

COOK'S NOTES

RICH IN ESSENTIAL FATS

LOW ALLERGY RATING
(wheat/dairy/egg/yeast-free)

V VEGETARIAN

MAKE WITH YOUR CHILD

SUITABLE FOR FREEZING

100g (4oz) good quality dark chocolate, broken into rough
chunks

2 tbsp tahini or unsalted hazelnut butter (from health-food
stores)

50g (2oz) oats

50g (2oz) mixed unsalted nuts, roughly chopped

50g (2oz) desiccated coconut

50g (2oz) pumpkin seeds

A good tbsp of ground or cracked flaxseeds (linseeds)

Ground cinnamon and/or ground ginger, to taste (optional)

1 Melt the chocolate then stir in the tahini. Place ten paper
  cake cases on a baking sheet.
2 Mix in the dry ingredients until evenly coated then spoon
  into the cake cases and chill until set.

Marzipan Shapes

A favourite with children, as they can indulge their love of playing with food to make the almond paste into shapes such as fruits, footballs, flowers, letters or faces. It is best to avoid the additive-ridden food colourings and sugary cake decorations – you can decorate the shapes with nuts or seeds such as finely chopped almonds or hazelnuts, or dip the shapes into a little melted chocolate and leave to set. This simple, no-cook recipe is sugar-free and the almonds contain calcium and magnesium for healthy bones, whereas the eggs provide memory-boosting protein and zinc, and mood- and energy-enhancing B vitamins. You will have some egg whites left over from the recipe; keep them in the fridge and add to omelettes for a very light, high-protein omelette (use two whole eggs and one white per person).

65g (2¼oz) ground almonds

15g (½oz) xylitol

2 free range or organic egg yolks

1 Mix all the ingredients together to form a smooth paste. Taste to check the flavour – you can add a little more xylitol for extra sweetness if needed.

2 Make into shapes and place on a plate or baking sheet. Store in the fridge for up to 1 week.

MAKES ABOUT 6

Parent's verdict: 'Easy to make, fun to do with children.'

Tested by: Hope, aged 10. Verdict: 'Fun to make, and it was nice and yummy.'

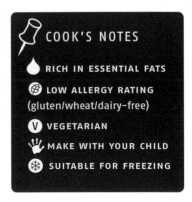

COOK'S NOTES

💧 RICH IN ESSENTIAL FATS

Ⓢ LOW ALLERGY RATING (gluten/wheat/dairy-free)

Ⓥ VEGETARIAN

✋ MAKE WITH YOUR CHILD

❄ SUITABLE FOR FREEZING

 HEALTH NOTE

Because this recipe contains raw egg, always choose organic, or at the very least free range, eggs to reduce the likelihood of salmonella contamination, and do not serve to pregnant women, very young children, the elderly or infirm.

Drinks

Don't undo all your hard work at mealtimes by giving your child sugar- and additive-laden drinks, which can lead to hyperactivity. The obvious alternative is water, but most children find this understandably dull when compared with the lurid, fizzing concoctions that are marketed to them. We have therefore come up with some delicious drinks that look as good as they taste.

You can make your own fizzy drinks by adding sparkling mineral water to fruit juice or fruit juice concentrates (with no added sugar). Do make sure you use naturally sparkling water, however, and not carbonated, as this erodes tooth enamel. Pure fruit juice can also be diluted with a little water to provide a low-sugar drink (if your child is used to highly flavoured juice and squashes start off with just a splash of water and gradually increase until it is half water, half juice to let their taste buds adapt). See the note on Choosing Fruit Juices (on page 59) for advice on how to interpret the labels of fruit juices and drinks. Fruit smoothies are an easy way to get children to eat more fruit and they can have great fun experimenting with different flavours. Try the recipes in the Breakfast section on page 65, and our Tropical Smoothie here.

 XYLITOL

We use xylitol in several recipes in this chapter. When first using xylitol, increase your daily intake gradually to allow the body to adjust, as large quantities can have a laxative effect. Don't let your child go berserk sweetening their cereal, puddings or drinks with xylitol – they may get a runny tummy as a result. Used in moderation it is a healthy way to include sweet treats in your diet. Do not give to very young children (under two), however, as it is important to get high-calorie, nutrient-dense foods into them as their stomachs are small.

 FASCINATING FACT

Fizzy drinks get their fizz from a substance called phosphoric acid. The body uses calcium to neutralise this acid so that it doesn't damage us. This calcium comes from our bones. Choose organic fizzy drinks, which do not contain phosphoric acid, to avoid weakening bones and increasing the risk of osteoporosis.

Lemonade

Parent's verdict: 'Really nice – no contest with commercial lemonade!'

This lemonade is sugar-free and contains plenty of vitamin C from the freshly squeezed lemon juice.

juice of ½ lemon (1 tbsp)

2 tsp xylitol, or to taste

200ml (just under 7fl oz) naturally sparkling mineral water

slice of lemon, to decorate

Stir all the ingredients together until the xylitol dissolves. Serve with ice and a slice of lemon.

SERVES 1 (TALL GLASS)

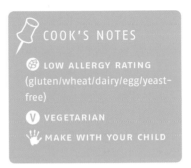

COOK'S NOTES

LOW ALLERGY RATING (gluten/wheat/dairy/egg/yeast-free)

V VEGETARIAN

MAKE WITH YOUR CHILD

Strawberry Fizz

Both strawberries and lemons are rich sources of vitamin C and this juice is very refreshing and utterly delicious. This recipe also works with raspberries.

100g (3½oz) (about 5) strawberries

juice of ½ lemon (1 tbsp)

2 tsp xylitol, or to taste

100ml (just over 3fl oz) naturally sparkling mineral water

2 strawberries, to decorate

SERVES 1 (SHORT GLASS)

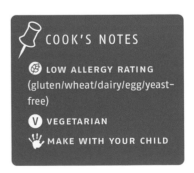

COOK'S NOTES

LOW ALLERGY RATING (gluten/wheat/dairy/egg/yeast-free)

V VEGETARIAN

MAKE WITH YOUR CHILD

1 Using a hand-held blender or a liquidiser, blend the strawberries and lemon juice until smooth. Stir in the xylitol until it has dissolved.
2 Mix in the mineral water and check the sweetness – add a little more xylitol if preferred. Serve chilled with ice and 2 strawberries in the glass.

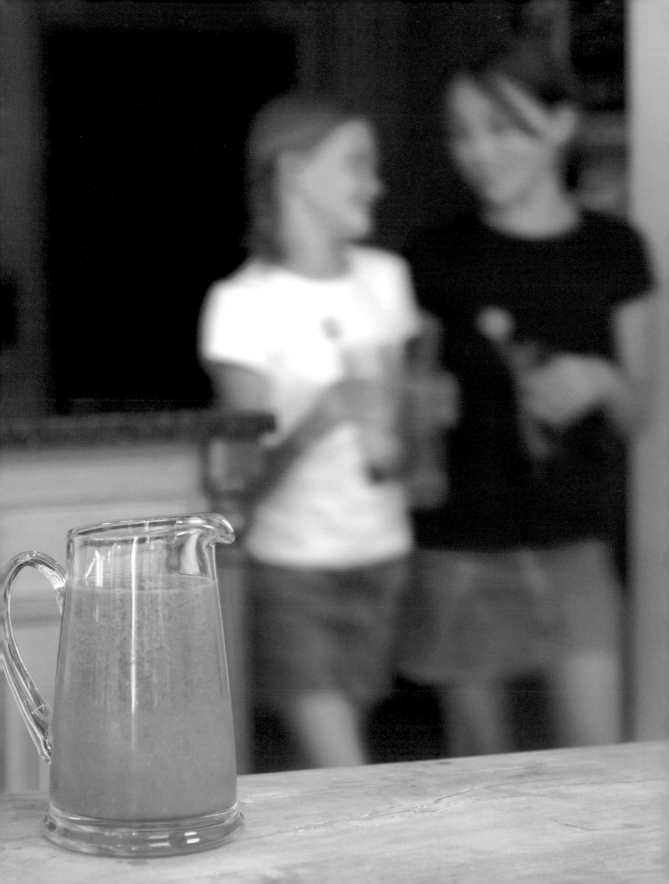

Watermelon Whizz

With its high water content, watermelon is perhaps the most refreshing of summer fruits. It is also very rich in beta-carotene, which keeps eyes and skin healthy. Keep the seeds in, as they blend completely into the smoothie and are packed with vitamin E.

medium slice of watermelon, about 200g (7oz) rindless weight

Blend the watermelon flesh, seeds and all, until smooth. Serve with ice or blend the ice with the watermelon for an instant chilled juice.

SERVES 1 (SHORT GLASS)

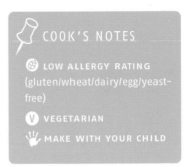

COOK'S NOTES

☻ LOW ALLERGY RATING (gluten/wheat/dairy/egg/yeast-free)

Ⓥ VEGETARIAN

✋ MAKE WITH YOUR CHILD

Tropical Smoothie

This makes a good liquid snack when it is too hot to want to eat. Bananas are excellent for the digestion and the fat from coconut is used as energy rather than being stored as fat. Add some strawberries to give this extra colour.

1 banana
150ml (¼ pint) coconut milk (shake the can before opening)
3 ice cubes

Blend all the ingredients together and drink immediately.

SERVES 1 (SHORT GLASS)

Parent's verdict: 'Just brilliant – we start every day with a smoothie now.'

 FASCINATING FACT

A 500ml (18fl oz) bottle of a leading brand of diluted blackcurrant squash contains the same amount of sugar as four tubes of chewy fruit sweets (that's 14½ teaspoons).

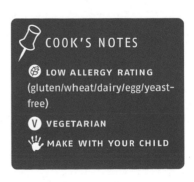

COOK'S NOTES

☻ LOW ALLERGY RATING (gluten/wheat/dairy/egg/yeast-free)

Ⓥ VEGETARIAN

✋ MAKE WITH YOUR CHILD

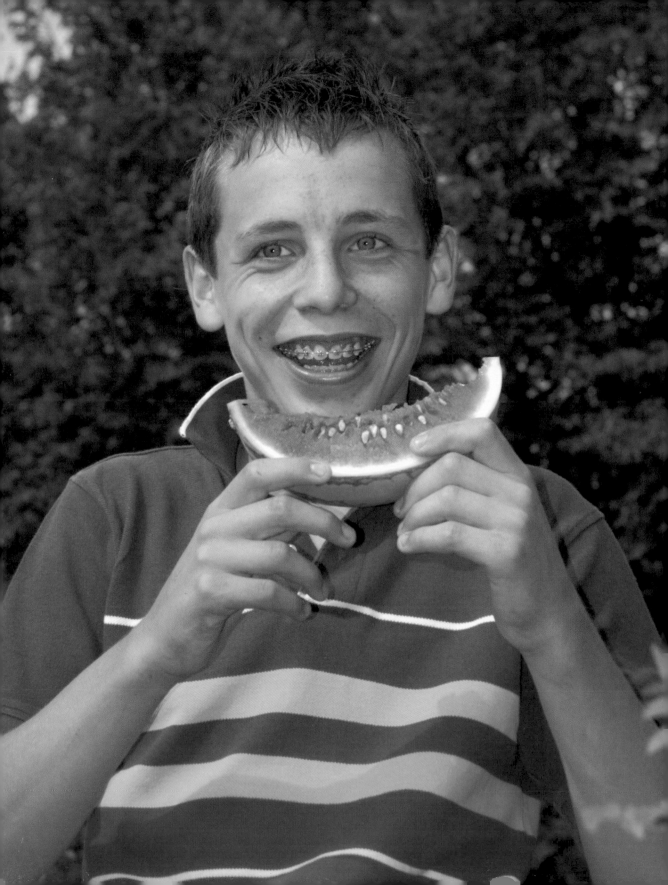

Eating Out

Now that you know the rules for healthy eating, you should be able to navigate your way around a menu without too many problems. Simply apply the same guidelines that you have been following at home, to make sure that your child's meal contains protein (such as meat, fish, eggs, beans or nuts) plus fruit or vegetables, and try to go for wholegrains such as brown rice rather than white versions if possible.

* Remember that restaurant portions of carbohydrates are normally much bigger than you would serve at home, so don't make your child finish everything on their plate if they have been presented with a bucketful of pasta or mounds of chips or mashed potato. Children's menus are usually the least healthy of all, featuring permutations of pizza, chips, nuggets and beans, so if necessary ask for a smaller portion of a dish from the standard menu. Order a large mixed salad or extra vegetables for everyone to pick at, and if your child will eat olives, ask for a bowl of these instead of white bread.

* Keep the GL of a pizza low by ordering a thin crust, or get one pizza to split between the table and fill up on other, healthier options as well. For toppings, steer your child towards extra vegetables and lean meat (such as chicken or fish) instead of those that are high in cheese – most restaurants will happily reduce the amount of cheese they use, or omit it entirely and simply add extra tomato sauce and toppings.

* Choose tomato- rather than cream- or cheese-based sauces, to avoid saturated fat and dairy products.

* If you are staying in a hotel and your child has particular food allergies, such as wheat or dairy products, inform the hotel in advance so that they can make sure they have suitable supplies available. It is also worth carrying a packet of oatcakes with you for when you are out and can find nothing available except bread and wheat-based bread products.

* If you are having a day out or going shopping keep plenty of healthy snacks to hand so that when your child is starving you can get some fruit and nuts or a healthy cereal bar out of your bag, to keep their blood sugar balanced and avoid sugar cravings and tantrums, instead of resorting to the lure of fast food or sweets, chocolate or fizzy drinks.

Chart Your Child's Progress

You should notice improvements to your child's physical and mental well-being after a week or so of improving their diet. Be prepared for a few days' cold turkey as you wean them off sugar, salt and additives, but after that their concentration, energy levels, mood and behaviour should all benefit.

	Week 1	Week 2	Week 3	Week 4
Sleep				
Mood				
Concentration				
Memory (school test results can help you score this)				
Sociability				
Physical energy				
Mental energy (score low for hyperactivity)				
Anxiety or nervousness				

This chart allows you to monitor the changes in your child over an eight-week period of following the dietary recommendations and recipes in this book. Each week give your child a score out of ten for each category and note any particular issues, success or achievements:

Week 5	Week 6	Week 7	Week 8	
				Sleep
				Mood
				Concentration
				Memory (school test results can help you score this)
				Sociability
				Physical energy
				Mental energy (score low for hyperactivity)
				Anxiety or nervousness

Recommended Reading

Burney, L., *Boost Your Child's Immune System*, Piatkus, 2003

Child, S., *An A–Z of Child Health: A Nutritional Approach*, Argyll, 2002

Cousins, Barbara, *Cooking Without*, HarperCollins, 2000

Holford, P., *The Holford Low-GL Diet*, Piatkus, 2004

Holford, P., *The New Optimum Nutrition Bible*, Piatkus, 2005

Holford, P. and Braly, J., *Hidden Food Allergies*, Piatkus, 2005

Holford, P. and Colson, D., *Optimum Nutrition for your Child's Mind*, Piatkus, 2005

Holford, P. and Lawson, S., *Optimum Nutrition Before During and After Pregnancy*, Piatkus, 2004

Holford, P. and McDonald Joyce, F., *The Holford Low-GL Diet Cookbook*, Piatkus, 2005

Holford, P., and Ridgeway, J. *The Optimum Nutrition Cookbook*, Piatkus, 2000

Richardson, Dr Alex, *They Are What You Feed Them*, Thorsons, 2006

Wigmore, A., *The Sprouting Book*, Avery, 1986

Resources

Allergy and homocysteine testing

Food allergy testing is best done under the guidance of a nutritional therapist or allergy testing specialist. YorkTest Laboratories offer a home-test kit for food allergy (IgG ELISA) and homocysteine testing. With this you can take your own pinprick blood sample and return it to the lab for analysis. This test identifies if you have any food allergies to 113 foods, including gluten and gliadin. Contact FREEPOST NEA5 243, York YO19 5ZZ, freephone 0800 074 6185 or visit www.yorktest.com.

Organic and allergy-free food service

A web- and mail-order shop for healthy foods, ranging from organic food to cruelty-free toiletries and environmentally friendly cleaning products. It is particularly useful for sourcing allergy-friendly ingredients for special diets, and delivers nation-wide. Order online at www.goodnessdirect.co.uk or call 0871 871 6611.

Meat

An internet search for 'mail-order meat' will bring up lots of suppliers that offer nationwide delivery, or look at your local farmers' market for local suppliers.

Salt alternatives

The average person gets far too much sodium because we eat too much salt (sodium chloride) and salted foods, and not enough potassium and magnesium, found in fruit and vegetables. Not all salt, however, is bad for you. Solo Low Sodium Sea Salt contains 60 per cent less sodium and is high in the essential minerals magnesium and potassium. Their 200g reusable shaker is sold in the UK, Ireland, Spain, Netherlands, Singapore, Hong Kong, Japan, Bahrain, Saudi Arabia, United Arab Emirates, Jordan, Baltic States and the United States of America. Visit their website www.soloseasalt.com for more information or call their international help line on +44 845 130 4568.

ABOUT THE FOOD FOR THE BRAIN FOUNDATION

A non-profit educational project, The Food for the Brain Foundation was created by a group of nutritionists, doctors, psychiatrists, psychologists, teachers and scientists to promote the link between nutrition and mental health. It aims to promote awareness of the link between learning, behaviour, mental health and nutrition; and to educate and provide educational material to children, parents, teachers, schools, the public, the catering industry, health professionals and the government.

Our vision is to create a future where the awareness of the importance of optimum nutrition for mental health is understood by all, and implemented by many; where:

* Babies are optimally nourished for brain development during pregnancy and infancy.
* Nurseries, schools and universities actively encourage optimum nutrition for brain function.
* Governments encourage optimum nutrition to promote learning and prevent behavioural and mental-health problems.
* Correcting nutritional imbalances is a first-line procedure in the treatment of mental-health problems.
* The public has easy access to information about optimum nutrition for mental health.

YOUR CHILD'S QUESTIONNAIRE
When you complete the Food for the Brain online questionnaire (www.foodfor thebrain.org) you'll receive personalised guidance on what your child really needs to maximise their performance. It's well worth doing.

As much as we would like to help transform every school in Britain, including yours, the reality is that it costs money. Food for the Brain is a charity and the two school projects mentioned at the beginning of this book have only been possible due to hundreds of small donations from people like you (if you'd like to make a donation visit www.foodforthebrain.org). We are hoping to receive funds to transform many other schools. If you would like your school to be one of these please ask the head to visit www.foodforthebrain.org and register their school's interest. Even if your school isn't selected, or doesn't have the means to pay, the website contains all kinds of resources they can use in their school, free of charge; for example, to help transform breakfast clubs, packed lunches, school menus and snack policy.

Visit www.foodforthebrain.org to become a friend.

Xylitol

Xylitol is a sugar alternative that does not upset blood sugar balance, making it ideal for dieters and diabetics. It can be used in exactly the same quantities as sugar in hot drinks, cooking, or sprinkled over fruit or cereals, and is available from selected Sainsbury's, Tesco, Waitrose, Holland and Barrett, and independent health-food stores as well as by mail-order from www.healthproductsforlife.com.

IN THE PINK

p_{the}ink
cooking for optimum nutrition

Fiona McDonald Joyce's specialist nutrition and cooking consultancy for individuals and corporate clients, including recipe and menu development and analysis, lectures, demonstrations and food, and health writing. If you would like more information or to book Fiona to appear at an event, please contact her at fiona@inthepink.co.uk or visit her website, www.inthepink.co.uk.

Mind and nutrition

The Brain Bio Centre is a London-based treatment clinic, part of the Food for the Brain Foundation, that puts the optimum nutrition approach into practice for people with mental-health problems, including learning difficulties, dyslexia, ADHD, autism, Alzheimer's, dementia, memory loss, depression, anxiety and schizophrenia.

For more information visit www.brainbiocentre. com or call 020 8832 9600.

The Institute for Optimum Nutrition (ION) offers a three-year foundation degree course in nutritional therapy that includes training in the optimum nutrition approach to mental health. There is a clinic, a list of nutrition practitioners across the UK, an information service and a quarterly journal – *Optimum Nutrition*.

Contact ION at Avalon House, 72 Lower Mortlake Road, Richmond TW9 2JY, UK, or call 020 8614 7800 or visit www.ion.ac.uk.

To find a nutritional therapist near you who we recommend, visit www.patrickholford.com and click on 'consultations'.

Food and Behaviour Research is a charitable organisation dedicated both to advancing scientific research into the links between nutrition and human behaviour and to making the findings from such research available to the widest possible audience. They have an excellent website and a free e-news service. Sign up at www.fabresearch.org.

The Food and Mood Project aims to empower individuals to explore the relationship between diet, nutrition and emotional and mental health, and to share this information with others. They have a quarterly newsletter, put on conferences and work closely with Mind to help improve awareness of the nutrition link to mental-health problems.

For more information visit www.foodandmood. org.

ADHD/Hyperactivity

The Hyperactive Children's Support Group (HACSG) is a UK-based charity organisation that offers support and information to parents and professionals who wish to pursue a drug-free approach to treating ADHD. They help and support hyperactive children and their parents, conduct research, promote investigation into the incidence of hyper-activity in the UK, investigate its causes and treatments, and spread information concerning the condition. There are some local groups in the UK which have been started by the parents of hyper-active children. There are also contact parents who have offered to help newly joined members in their locality.

Contact HACSG at 71 Whyke Lane, Chichester, West Sussex PO19 2PD, UK, for all information, diet booklets, articles and general requests (enclose a stamped SAE). Or call 01243 551313, or visit www.hacsg.org.uk.

Autism

The National Autistic Society UK was founded in 1962 by parents frustrated by the lack of provision and support for children with autism and their carers, with the aim of encouraging a better understanding of autism and to pioneer specialist services for people with autism and those who care for them.

Contact the National Autistic Society UK at 393 City Road, London EC1V 1NG, UK, or call 020 7833 2299, or visit www.nas.org.uk.

Autism Research Institute (ARI), founded by Bernard Rimland PhD, is the hub of a worldwide network of parents and professionals concerned with autism. The only organisation of its kind, ARI was founded in 1967 to conduct and foster scientific research designed to improve the methods of diagnosing, treating and preventing autism. ARI also disseminates research findings to parents and others all over the world who are seeking help. The ARI data bank, the world's largest, contains nearly 25,000 detailed case histories of autistic children from over 60 countries.

Contact ARI at 4182 Adams Avenue, San Diego, California 92116, US, or visit www.autism.com/ari.

Product and Supplement Directory

Supplements

Multivitamin and mineral supplements

The best multivitamin formula, based on optimum nutrition levels, is BioCare's Optimum Nutrition for Kids. Very young children can take Ola Loa (from www.drinkyourvitamins.com) – a multi in a sachet that is mixed with water to make a pleasant-tasting, slightly effervescent drink.

BioCare makes an excellent range of liquid mineral and vitamin products. These can be added in drop form to other drinks and food. In addition, BioCare makes a couple of vitamin-C powder products, which provide additional minerals and can also be added to drinks or food.

Essential fats and fish-oil supplements

The most important omega-3 fats are DHA and EPA, the richest source being cod liver oil. The most important omega-6 fat is GLA, the richest source being borage (also known as starflower) oil. Our favourite is BioCare's Omega Chews, which provides a highly concentrated mix of DHA, EPA and GLA.

Equazen's Eye Q range includes capsules, liquids and strawberry chews. It can be found in most supermarkets and high-street chemists.

Vegetarian options do not provide DHA and EPA directly, only the precursors – so they're not our first choice for these omega-3s. But if you want to go for vegetarian options, choose BioCare's Microcell Essential Fatty Acids.

Brain support and phospholipid supplements

Additional brain nutrients include phospholipids such as phosphatidyl choline and phosphatidyl serine, and pyroglutamate and DMAE. Phosphatidyl choline (PC) can be found in lecithin granules, which are a pleasant-tasting addition to breakfast foods. BioCare's Brain Food Formula contains a blend of these brain-support nutrients, plus some ginkgo.

Company directory

UK

The following companies produce good-quality supplements that are widely available in the UK.

Totally Nourish is an online shop that stocks most of the supplements and other products mentioned above, including Xylosweet (the sugar substitute xylitol). You can order from them directly from the website www.totallynourish.com or by telephone on 0800 085 7749.

BioCare produces a wide range of nutritional and herbal supplements, including an excellent children's range, which is available in any good health-food shop. For your nearest supplier, call 0121 433 3727 or visit www.biocare.co.uk.

Solgar produces a wide range of nutritional and herbal supplements available in any good health-food shop. For your nearest supplier, call 01442 890355 or visit www.solgar.co.uk.

Outside the UK

South Africa Bioharmony produces a wide range of products in South Africa and other African countries. We recommend their Smart Kids chewable multivitamin. For details of your nearest supplier call 0860 888 339 or visit www.bioharmony.co.za.

Australia Solgar supplements are available in Australia. Contact Solgar on 1800 029 871 (free call) for your nearest supplier, or visit www.solgar.com.au. Another good brand is Blackmores.

New Zealand BioCare products are available in New Zealand. Contact Aurora Natural Therapies, 445 Dillons Point Road, RD3, Blenheim, Marlborough, New Zealand, or call (64) 3578 1236/(64) 27449 8573, or visit www.aurora.org.nz.

Singapore BioCare and Solgar products are available in Singapore. Contact Essential Living on 6276 1380 for your nearest supplier or visit www.essliv.com.

Notes

1 Department of Health, Summary of intelligence on obesity (2004), www.dh.gov.uk/assetRoot/04/09/49/76/040949 76.pdf

2 www.educationworld.com/a_issues/ issues148a.shtml

3 Biederman, J. and Faraone, S. V., 'Attention-deficit Hyperactivity Disorder', *Lancet*, Vol 366 (2005), pp. 237–48

4 Baird, G. et al., *Lancet*, Vol 368 (2006), pp. 210–15

5 Borjel, A. K. *et al.*, 'Plasma homocysteine levels, MTHFR polymorphisms 677C>T, 1298A>C, 1793G>A, and school achievement in a population sample of Swedish children', paper presented at Homocysteine Metabolism, 5th International Conference, Milan (Italy), 26–30 June, 2005

6 Penland, J., Experimental Biology conference, San Diego, 4 April 2005 (pending publication)

7 Benton, D. and Roberts, G., 'Effect of vitamin and mineral supplementation on intelligence of school children', *Lancet*, Vol 1(1988), pp. 140–3

8 Benton, D., ' Micro-nutrient supplementation and the intelligence of school children', *Neuroscience and Behavioural Reviews*, Vol 25 (2001), pp. 297-309

9 Young, E. *et al.*, 'A population study of food intolerance', *Lancet*, Vol 343, (1994), pp. 1127–9

10 *Effective Allergy Practice*, British Society for Allergy and Environmental Medicine (1984)

11 Randolph, T., 'Allergy as a causative factor of fatigue, irritability and behaviour problems of children', *J Pediatr*, Vol 31 (1947), p. 560

12 Rowe, A., 'Allergic toxemia and fatigue', *Annals of Allergy*, Vol 17 (1959), p. 9

13 Spccr, F., (cd.), 'Etiology: Foods', in *Allergy of the Nervous System*, Charles Thomas (1970)

14 Campbell, M., 'Neurologic manifestations of allergic disease', *Annals of Allergy*, Vol 31 (1973), p. 485

15 Hall, K., 'Allergy of the nervous system: A review', *Annals of Allergy*, Vol 36 (1976), pp. 49–64

16 Pippere, V., 'Some varieties of food intolerance in psychiatric patients', *Nutritional Health*, Vol 3 (3) (1984), pp. 125–36

17 Boris, M. D. and Mandel, F. S., 'Foods and additives are common causes of the attention deficit hyperactive disorder in children', *Annals of Allergy*, Vol 72 (1994), pp. 462–468

18 Carter, C. M. et al., 'Effects of a few food diet in attention deficit disorder', *Archives of Disease in Childhood*, Vol 69 (1993), pp. 564–8

Index

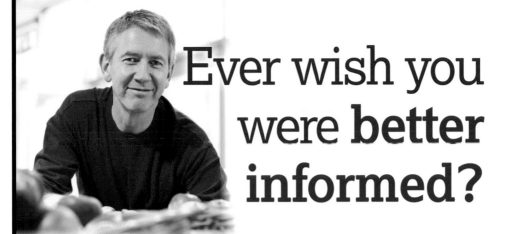

Ever wish you were **better** informed?

Join my 100% Health Club today and you'll receive:

- ✔ My newsletter, plus Special Reports on vital health topics

- ✔ Immediate access to hundreds of health articles and special reports.

- ✔ Have your questions answered in our Members Only blogs.

- ✔ Save money on supplements, books and other health products.

- ✔ Save up to £50 on Patrick Holford's **100% Health Workshop**.

- ✔ Become part of a community of like-minded people and help others.

JOIN TODAY at **www.patrickholford.com**

66 Being a member has transformed my life, and that of many of my family and friends. Patrick's information is always spot on and really practical. My member benefits and discounts save me much more than the subscription. Being a member is a must if you want to be and stay healthy. 99

Joyce Taylor

100%Health®
Weekend Intensive
The workshop that works.

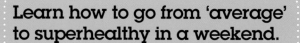

Learn how to go from 'average' to superhealthy in a weekend.

Do YOU want to:

✔ Take control of your own health?

✔ Master your weight?

✔ Turn back the clock?

✔ Prevent and reverse disease?

✔ Transform your diet, your health and your life?

Discover the **8 secrets of optimum living** - and put them into action with your own individualised personal health and fitness programme with **Patrick Holford**.

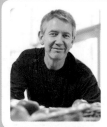

"You can wake up full of energy, with a clear mind and balanced mood, never gain weight and stay disease free. Having worked with over 60,000 people I know what changes are going to most rapidly transform how you feel."

Patrick Holford

Thousands of people have transformed their health.

Why not become one of them?
Find out more at **www.patrickholford.com**

100%Health® is the registered trademark of Holford & Associates